About the authors

Caroline Walker is a nutritionist. She studied biology at Queen Elizabeth College, London University, and nutrition at the School of Hygiene and Tropical Medicine. She has worked at the Medical Research Council epidemiology unit in South Wales, and at the Dunn Clinical Nutrition Centre, Cambridge. She is Secretary of the Coronary Prevention Group, and is responsible for the heart disease prevention programme in City and Hackney health district. She was Secretary of the working group responsible to Professor Philip James that produced the NACNE report.

Geoffrey Cannon is a writer and editor. He studied Philosophy, Psychology and Physiology at Balliol College, Oxford, and was a founder member of the editorial staff of *New Society*. From 1980 to 1983 he was an Assistant Editor at *The Sunday Times*. He writes a monthly column for *Running* magazine, and for *New Health* magazine of which he is Consultant Editor. He is author of *Dieting Makes You Fat* with Hetty Einzig. As a writer, his chief interest is the relationship between food and health, and he wrote the *Sunday Times* features that revealed the existence of the NACNE report.

The Food Scandal

*What's Wrong with the British Diet
and How to Put it Right*

CAROLINE WALKER and
GEOFFREY CANNON

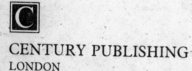

CENTURY PUBLISHING
LONDON

To Philip James and Jerry Morris

Where there is no vision the people perish.   Proverbs 29:18

Copyright © Caroline Walker & Geoffrey Cannon 1984, 1985

All rights reserved

First published in Great Britain in 1984
by Century Publishing Co. Ltd

First published as a paperback in 1985
by Century Publishing Co. Ltd,
Portland House
12–13 Greek Street, London W1V 5LE

British Library Cataloguing in Publication Data

Walker, Caroline
  The Food Scandal
  1. Diet – Great Britain
  I. Title   II. Cannon, Geoffrey
  613.2'0941   RA784

  ISBN 0 7126 0785 4

Typeset by Avocet, Aylesbury, Bucks
Printed in Great Britain in 1985 by
The Guernsey Press Co. Ltd,
Guernsey, Channel Islands.

Acknowledgements

Acknowledgement of the doctors whose work has informed us would begin with Hippocrates. It is only recently that medicine has lost touch with the first fundamental statement about food and health, which is: you are what you eat.

Nor can we acknowledge individually all the authorities whose findings are crowding into leading medical and scientific journals, and showing repeatedly that the quality of our lives depends on the quality of our food.

This new edition owes much to the many people in government, science and industry who have supported, criticised, advised, informed or warned us, since first publication in the summer of 1984. Some of them are acknowledged below.

While responsibility for this book and the judgments in it are ours, our thanks go to Dr Keith Ball, Dr Walter Barker, Professor Norman Blacklock, Dr Denis Burkitt, Dr David Buss, Professor John Catford, Dr Michael Church, Professor Michael Crawford, Professor John Dickerson, Wendy Doyle, Professor John Farquhar, Walter Fleiss, John Forsyth, Dr John Garrow, Barbara Griggs, Dr Walter Hare, Dr Kenneth Heaton, Professor Mark Hegsted, Dorothy Hollingsworth, Dr Sandra Hunt, Professor Philip James, Leslie Kenton, William Laing, Bob Laird, Dr Tim Lang, Dr Alan Long, Alistair Mackie, Dr Donald McLaren, Professor Jerry Morris, Dr Brian Nicholls, Professor Michael Oliver, Professor Ralph Paffenbarger, Dr Sheldon Reiser, John Rivers, Christopher Robbins, David Roberts, Professor Geoffrey Rose, Maggie Sanderson, Professor Aubrey Sheiham, Helena Sheiham, Dr

Hugh Sinclair, Professor Alwyn Smith, Dr David Southgate, Professor Jeremiah Stamler, Dr Hugh Trowell, Professor Stewart Truswell, Colin Tudge, Dr Richard Turner, David Walker, Professor Peter Wood, Arthur Wynn, Margaret Wynn, Dr Walter Yellowlees, and Professor John Yudkin.

After the pioneering work of Sir Robert McCarrison, Lord Boyd Orr, Sir Jack Drummond and Surgeon-Captain T. L. Cleave, the present leaders of the new public health movement, who – if anyone can – will make Britain once again a healthy nation, include Sir Douglas Black, Sir Richard Doll, Sir Francis Avery Jones, and Professor Thomas McKeown. Thanks to them and others, any voice raised is not crying in a wilderness.

Professional support has been given by Don Berry, Features Editor of *The Sunday Times*, Nicholas Wapshott, first of *The Times*, now Features Editor of *The Observer*, and Felicity Lawrence, Editor of *New Health*; by our agent, Deborah Rogers; and by our publishers Anthony Cheetham, Peter Roche, Gail Rebuck, Sarah Wallace and Susan Lamb. We would also like to thank Neil Biggs, James Crocker, Jonathan Crystal, Mick Finnerty, Dr Ken Grant, Carole Hobson, Ted Key, Richard Marshall, Karen North, Miranda Page-Wood, Penny Phipps, Richard Sykes and Leslie Webber.

Caroline Walker
Geoffrey Cannon
April 1985

Contents

The Story of the Food Scandal

CONFUSED MESSAGES. THE MCGOVERN REPORT.
FOOD POLICY: WHO DECIDES? NACNE UNDERMINED.
ADDED VALUE: FOR WHOM? A PUBLIC HEALTH SCANDAL.

'Nutrition in Britain is generally good.' That is official: the latest word of the government on the subject, issued by the Department of Health in 1981. It is neither a new nor a Conservative message: word for word, it repeats the DHSS statement made under a Labour government in 1969.

It is nice not to worry about food. Politicians have got plenty on their plates already. Doctors are not taught nutrition. Agriculture is a success story. Industry wants to keep the wheels of commerce turning. Everybody likes to relax over a meal. The story for the past forty years in Britain has been that any public health problem caused by food is marginal. That is what we have been brought up to believe. We have been misled.

In the 1960s the thrill had gone from the study of human nutrition. Most good British scientists in the field were studying protein and energy malnutrition in the Third World. Britain had been solved. After all, British children had their free milk and balanced meals at school, and the national food supply was plentiful. Mass outbreaks of queues or food poisoning were rare.

In 1970 the Conservatives came to power, and Margaret Thatcher became notorious, as minister responsible for education, with what became the Education (Milk) Act (1971). This withdrew the free supply of milk to schoolchildren over 7 years old. Mrs Thatcher's reputation as 'milk snatcher' was not really justified; she was continuing a process begun by the previous Labour government. However, milk was (and is) an emotional subject; and Mrs Thatcher attracted more criticism in 1971 when the price of school meals was raised from 9p to 12p.

Confused Messages

Would the health of the nation suffer when children deprived of school milk grew up? Just how vital was cow's milk, anyway? Did children still need the protection of subsidized and 'balanced' school meals? These and other questions rippled the calm pool of human nutrition. Under the surface there were other eddies and cross currents, known to those in government with responsibility for the nation's health. Rickets had reappeared, largely, it was thought, among the Asian community. People seemed to be getting fatter; was this true and did it matter? Obviously obesity was diet-related: what about heart disease? And, certainly, the British teeth were in a mess.

Messages directed to the public by the food industry, the media and the slimming industry were becoming more confusing and contradictory in the early 1970s. This alone would not have concerned policy-makers in government, were it not for the fact that they and their scientific advisors were in a muddle too. What was good food, what was bad food, and, once again, did it matter? There were practical problems. What should health visitors be instructed to tell mothers about milk? Should doctors and dentists give advice to their fat and carious patients? What, in a word, was the line?

It is in such circumstances, in Britain, that committees are formed. Accordingly, Sir Keith Joseph, then minister responsible for health, set up a working party, of people from the DHSS, from the Health Education Council (funded by the DHSS) and from the British Nutrition Foundation (funded by the food industry). In 1978, five years after Sir Keith's initiative, the working party recommended that 'there is an urgent need for a point of reference that would provide simple and accurate information on nutrition.' Accordingly, the National Advisory Committee on Nutrition Education was formed on 16 July 1979. It became known as NACNE.

Under the chairmanship of Professor J. N. (Jerry) Morris, a veteran of many committees on matters of public health, NACNE 'set to work with a will' (in Morris's words) but soon lost momentum; the reason being 'that it would not be possible to make progress with its task unless the conflicting advice being offered on many sides on what is a healthful diet was first resolved.' You cannot, after all, give simple and accurate information about food and health if you don't know what you are talking about.

Again in Morris's words, 'an authoritative statement of the present consensus over the whole field' was needed. So at a meeting held on 9 May 1980 the vice-chairman of NACNE, Dr Philip James, was asked to form a working party and compile such a statement. A paper on general principles was agreed at this meeting. It stated that objectives were to include cuts in the national consumption of sugar, animal and vegetable fats and (perhaps) salt, and the promotion of bread, fresh vegetables and fruit. A cut in national alcohol consumption was also an objective.

It was agreed that 'clear and simple messages were necessary, and unambiguous advice that could be put into practice by the public.' It was also agreed that the chief sources for Dr James's report should be expert reports already published by the DHSS, the Royal College of Physicians, and such bodies.

Once the work was done and the report agreed, industry

could then be approached through the British Nutrition Foundation, and agreement sought for 'slow change'.

The McGovern Report

While the pre-NACNE working party was deliberating on nutrition education in Britain, a committee of the United States Senate, chaired by the former Presidential candidate George McGovern, was working towards a report called *Dietary Goals for the United States*, published in February 1977. With all-party backing from a committee that included such grandees as Hubert Humphrey, Edward Kennedy, Charles Percy and Robert Dole, the McGovern report stated

> The simple fact is that our diets have changed radically within the past 50 years, with great and very harmful effects on our health . . . Too much fat, too much sugar or salt, can be and are linked directly to heart disease, cancer, obesity and stroke, among other killer diseases . . . Those of us within government have an obligation to acknowledge this. The public wants some guidance, wants to know the truth.

And Republican senator Percy added 'without government and industry commitment to good nutrition, the American people will continue to eat themselves to bad health . . . Our national health depends on how well and how quickly government and industry respond.'

Dr Mark Hegsted, Professor of Nutrition at Harvard Medical School, chief scientific advisor to the McGovern committee, added a note to the report: 'The diet we eat today was not planned or developed for any particular purpose. It is a happenstance related to our affluence, the productivity of our farmers and the activities of our food industry' and he went on to make a key statement:

> What are the risks associated with eating less meat, less fat, less saturated fat, less cholesterol, less sugar, less salt, and more fruits, vegetables, unsaturated fat and cereal products – especially whole

grain cereals? There are none that can be identified and important benefits can be expected. Heart disease, cancer, diabetes and hypertension are the diseases that kill us. They are epidemic in our population . . . We have an obligation . . . to assist the public in making the correct food choices. To do less is to avoid our responsibility.

After a furious debate during 1977, involving pressure groups representing both consumers on the one side, and food manufacturers on the other, a debate in which the American nation as a whole was involved, a second edition of the McGovern report was issued in December of that year. It remains available from government bookshops in America. It includes targets for a healthy diet, with less fats, saturated fats, sugars and salt; and much more 'complex carbohydrates' from whole food high in fibre, vitamins and minerals, together with naturally occurring sugars (from fruit and other sources). These targets were precise: for example, consumption of saturated fats should drop to 10 per cent of total calories (from an estimated 16 per cent) and processed, 'refined' sugars should also drop to 10 per cent of total calories (from an estimated 18 per cent).

With support from the US government departments of health and of agriculture, the McGovern report also made some estimates of the lives and money that could be saved, and health and welfare improved, by a national healthy diet. Of the many estimates, some stand out: a saving of 250,000 deaths a year from heart disease (a quarter of the total); a corresponding saving of $10 thousand million a year on treatment of heart disease and strokes; a 5 per cent increase in work productivity; and an average increase of 10 IQ points in children of low intelligence.

In America the fats, sugars and salt were in the fire. Human nutrition had once again become big stuff.

Food Policy: Who Decides?

Back in Britain, members of the NACNE committee and sub-committee with expert knowledge were of course well aware that the consensus of modern scientific thinking about food and health was reflected in the McGovern report. They were also aware that Americans were changing their food habits towards the goals recommended by McGovern, and that the rates of death and premature death from heart disease in the USA were dropping fast.

In 1981 Philip James, a nutritionist who is also a doctor of medicine, was deputy director of the Dunn Clinical Nutrition Centre in Cambridge. Over the weekend of 9–11 January, as charged by the NACNE committee, he brought together a sub-committee of ten doctors and nutritionists, to discuss how to proceed.

Some fundamental decisions were taken at the Cambridge weekend meeting, which remained key to NACNE thinking. In particular, the learning of the 1930s and 1940s, which had become the official policy dogma of the 1960s and 1970s in Britain, was contradicted as unhelpful, irrelevant, misleading, out of date, or just plain wrong. For instance:

- The priority should be the health of the nation as a whole, not (as officially thought) avoidance of deficiency diseases by isolated 'special groups'.

- The problem is the British diet as a whole, high in fats, sugars and salt, not (as officially agreed) the personal eating habits of people who 'overdid it'.

- The plan for action should be to change the eating habits of the nation as a whole, not (as officially hoped) merely the habits of those who were already ill or 'at risk'.

To quote a later draft of the report: 'the consensus of medical opinion is that the population should not be consuming the type of diet currently eaten in Britain.'

This was of course already well known to DHSS civil servants and advisors. But in published documents the message was muted. For instance, *Eating for Health* remains the latest DHSS word on food and health for the lay reader. Obtainable at any HMSO bookshop, it has this to say about overweight: 'Food intake should not be greater than is necessary for energy expenditure. A practical way of ensuring this is not to become overweight for one's height.' And in general: 'the message is one of moderation. Enough is enough: more is not better and can be harmful.' Yes indeed!

One clear message in DHSS publications is that if you eat bad food and suffer as a result, that is your fault. The other current relevant booklet for the lay reader, *Prevention and Health: Everybody's Business* has this to say:

> The role of the health professions and of government is limited to ensuring that the public has access to such knowledge as is available about the importance of personal habit on health and that at the very least no obstacles are placed in the way of those who decide to act on that knowledge.

Apart from the irony in the last part of this underpunctuated passage, it points to what is perhaps the key difference between the policy proposed by the NACNE sub-committee, and the policy still, in 1985, followed by government. The implication of NACNE is that food and health is not principally an individual, but a national problem, and that

- The solution involves government taking a responsibility for a healthy food supply and not (as officially stated) assuming that as a nation we are now free to choose healthy food.

'Once the public know what is really in the food they buy, and the risks they run in eating it, there will be a revolution in the food industry', wrote Sir Woodrow Wyatt in *The Times*, on 17 November 1984. But what are the public being told? Here is *Eating for Health* again, on the quality of British food since the 1950s. 'The good effects on health have over-whelmingly exceeded any ill-effects.'

If you supposed that advice on food and health published by government is a summary of the most reliable and up-to-date scientific judgment, untouched by 'considerations of state', you would be wrong.

That is not how things work. Advice given to the DHSS or to the Ministry of Agriculture (MAFF) that is liable to cause political problems, is therefore liable to be redrafted, rewritten, suppressed, ignored or overturned.

Who are the expert DHSS and MAFF advisors? They are chosen by civil servants, to serve either on the DHSS 'COMA' committee (the initials are short for 'Committee on Medical Aspects of Food Policy') or else on the MAFF Food Advisory Committee (formed in November 1983 by the amalgamation of the rather more explicitly named Food Standards Committee, and the Food Additives and Contaminants Committee).

While the status of these committees is, formally, advisory, they are the source of government policy on food and health, including legislation on food labelling, standards and composition, in so far as any such policy has a scientific basis.

Industry always has a voice on these committees. Some MAFF sub-committees have strong industry representation. For example, that on Food Safety Research, due to report by 31 August 1985, includes men from Cadbury Schweppes, Unilever, Beechams and Whitbread, in a committee of ten. Food manufacturers are not directly represented on COMA panels but as often as not these include somebody from the industry-funded British Nutrition Foundation.

This is not to suggest that members of DHSS and MAFF committees give anything but their best advice. But it stands to reason that people who work for industry or who are paid by industry will have views harmonious with the interests of industry.

There again, a number of scientists with international

reputation, who are critical of the quality of the food manufactured and supplied in Britain, have not been invited by DHSS or MAFF officials to serve on advisory committees, although they may submit their views privately. These submissions are not published.

Members of DHSS and MAFF committees and sub-committees on food and health are required to sign the Official Secrets Act.

NACNE Undermined

The NACNE main committee had been set up in 1979 as a forum for representatives of government, science, industry and health education. When Dr James presented the first draft of his report, which he had completed early in 1981, there was uproar.

At a meeting of the full NACNE committee held on 4 March 1982, the DHSS representative claimed that Dr James and his group had exceeded their brief and that there was no justification for recommending that the British diet is too high in sugars or salt, or too low in fibre. The representative also said that the report failed to understand the DHSS concept of 'special' and 'at risk' groups, and that anyway Dr James had no right to present a document containing *ex-cathedra* statements.

Dr Michael Turner, one of the two representatives of the British Nutrition Foundation on NACNE, at first welcomed the report, in writing; but then in committee attacked it as a shoddy document which made recommendations to cut sugars and alcohol, for which there was no justification. John Wood of the Food and Drink Industries Council (now the Food and Drink Federation) sat by Dr Turner's side during the meeting, taking notes.

On 3 March 1981, a month before Dr James had completed his first draft, Michael Shersby MP put a Parliamentary Question to the DHSS saying, 'Will my Honourable Friend consider urgently the possibility of arranging for the Health Education Council to subcontract to the British Nutrition Foundation its responsibilities for health education?' The DHSS reply demurred. Michael Shersby was and is Director-General of the British Sugar Bureau (now the Sugar Bureau).

Dr James was asked to go away and think again, which he did, and a new draft, together with 87 references to the scientific literature, was presented on 3 November 1982. A number of bodies and individuals with special knowledge, notably of diet and heart disease, had been consulted, and a new World Health Organisation report on the prevention of heart disease had been incorporated.

Among the recommendations of the WHO expert committee, chaired by Professor Geoffrey Rose from London University, was the following:

> Emphasize: appropriately combined foods of plant origin: beans, cereal grains, vegetables (cooked and raw), and fruit (offering good-quality protein, low fat, low saturated fat, low cholesterol, low sodium, low refined sugar, high complex carbohydrates, high vitamins, minerals and fibre, and lower energy intake.

The second draft of what became known as the 'NACNE report' proposed a 15-year plan for change, saying

> If industry, including both the agricultural and food industry, recognizes at this stage that a consensus is emerging among expert medical groups and that a dietary change is being advocated for the general population, they can make plans in good time to achieve the adjustments suggested.

An Emerged Consensus

In fact, a global consensus (meaning general agreement) had already emerged. Between 1968 and 1978 twenty expert committee reports on heart disease prevention or, more generally, on dietary goals, had been published, from the USA, Canada, Germany, Holland, Norway, Sweden, Finland,

Australia, New Zealand and, indeed, Britain. All accepted that heart disease is diet-related. All proposed changes in diet. Almost all proposed targets. Most recommended a cut in fats consumption (16) and sugars consumption (14) for the general population. None had any enthusiasm for saturated fats or sugars.

Between 1978 and 1982 the pace quickened, and another 17 expert reports were published; after 1979, all recommended a cut in salt consumption for the general population.

The modern view on food and health is well summarized by Sir Richard Doll, a doctor of great distinction who has been Regius Professor of Medicine at Oxford University and director of research of the Imperial Cancer Research Fund, and who was jointly responsible for establishing the causal link between smoking and cancer. In October 1982, while Dr James was revising his document, Sir Richard stated in his Harveian Oration, a key speech given by and to leaders of the medical profesion:

> Whether the object is to avoid cancer, coronary heart disease, hypertension, diabetes, diverticular disease, duodenal ulcer, or constipation, there is a broad agreement among research workers that the type of diet that is least likely to cause disease is one that provides a high proportion of calories in whole grain cereals, vegetables and fruit; provides most of its animal protein in fish and poultry; limits the intake of fats, and, if oils are to be used, gives preference to liquid vegetable oils; includes very few dairy products, eggs, and little refined sugar.

What did the British Nutrition Foundation have to say? Dr Turner and Dr Juliet Gray, the two BNF members of the main NACNE committee, had been asked to state their views, which they had done, not in the form of any contribution to Dr James's report, but as a BNF publication published in May 1982, *Implementation of Dietary Guidelines: Obstacles and Opportunities*. With guidance from a working party of nine people other than BNF staff, including men from Beechams,

Rank Hovis McDougall, Tate & Lyle and Imperial Chemical Industries, Dr Turner and Dr Gray expressed worries about dietary guidelines.

Achieving a cut in fats consumption to 30 per cent of total energy, as recommended by the McGovern committee (and the NACNE report in draft) 'would require major changes in eating habits resulting in a diet of doubtful palatability' said Dr Turner and Dr Gray, citing as authority 'Thorn, 1980' which turned out to be a publication issued by the Butter Information Council, the propaganda arm of the butter industry. There again 'simply to say "let there be substantially less sugar or butter" for example, would have far-reaching economic implications worldwide'.

Nevertheless, the BNF publication did accept the medical consensus, that consumption of fats, sugars and salt should drop, and that consumption of cereals, vegetables and fruit should increase, for the sake of the national health.

Goals for Change

It is, however, one thing to say that we should consume less fat, sugars and salt. It is another thing to say just how much less fat, sugars and salt we should consume, and to set targets, with numbers.

Dr James was now Director of the Rowett Research Institute in Aberdeen, a post previously held by Britain's most influential nutritionist this century, John (later Lord) Boyd Orr. Professor James, as he now was, under pressure to make 'realistic and palatable' recommendations, was preparing a third draft of the NACNE report, which was ready in April 1983.

Short-term goals had now been introduced into the report. Given what it described as 'the intense commercial pressures to maintain sucrose intakes', the short-term goal for sugars was confined to a recommendation that consumption of confectionery and soft drinks be cut. The short-term goals were roughly one third of the long-term goals, and designed to be achieved by the individual 'while food manufacturers are making their more important reductions.'

In an attempt to break the deadlock, NACNE chairman Professor Morris wrote a preface to the third draft pointing out that 'every care was taken to consult the country's experts' and that

> The report that follows is in every sense a collaborative national effort. A particular effort has been made to state a programme for the 1980s which is scientifically based, feasible and worthwhile.

At least eleven of the eighteen members of the NACNE committee supported the report that Professor James had compiled; only the DHSS and BNF members, and Mr Wood, were definitely against it. But the DHSS committee members effectively had the power to veto the report. By now the DHSS had set up its own COMA committee, on 'Diet and Cardiovascular Disease', and proposed that NACNE should wait for COMA to report. Publicly the story was that a further wait was prudent. Privately, according to one civil servant, the intention was to 'torpedo' NACNE.

Big Noises from the BNF

What was the position of the British Nutrition Foundation? It was founded in 1967, with the brief of building bridges between industry, government and science, and of advising opinion formers and educators. While it has always been wholly funded by the food industry it has always stated that it is independent. In the words of BNF Secretary Paddy Victory: 'it is quite fatuous, and indeed insulting, to try to suggest that the eminent independent scientists on our Council and Advisory Committees would allow themselves to be manipulated, bullied or browbeaten by industry.'

Founders of the BNF include Rank Hovis McDougall, who now share 85 per cent of the British white bread market with

Allied Bakeries, and who also make 75 per cent of British table salt; Tate & Lyle, who monopolise the market for imported white sugar in Britain; and Beechams, the drug and food company whose branded products include Marmite, Bovril, Ribena and Lucozade. In 1985 these three firms all announced record annual profits, of £55.1 million, £69.2 million (annual) and £149.2 million (six months) respectively.

The food and chemical giants ICI and Unilever are also influential within the BNF. The industrial governors of the BNF, whose firms paid a £7,500 annual subscription, did not show any enthusiasm for the NACNE report between 1981 and 1983. Two letters addresssed to Dr Turner while he was preparing the BNF publication *'Dietary Guidelines'* give a clue to industry's attitude. Graham Harris of Mars Ltd wrote 'the necessity for and practicality of dietary guidelines in the UK at this time remains to be justified', and Mr E. F. Moss of the Quality Assurance department at Nestlé wrote: 'I am not in favour of nutritional labelling. There is no question but that industry will be faced with additional costs in order to carry this out.'

The aim of building bridges between industry and science is in principle admirable. In practice, as informed opinion has hardened against fats, saturated fats, sugars and salt, it has tended to be the fats and sugars manufacturers who have had most money to spend. Here is an example: an offer in a written letter from Dr Turner to a Medical Research Council Unit (not, in the event, taken up):

> I have been approached by the British Sugar Bureau with a view to establishing at their expense a proper scientific slimming trial in which 'sweets, treats and cheats' are permitted, i.e. from which sweet foods are not specifically excluded, as is usually the case.

In June 1984 Dr Alan Robertson of ICI, the BNF Chairman, was interviewed and asked for his view of the NACNE report. 'I am not prepared to say that we in Britain eat too much fat and sugar until I have the totality of the facts', he said; and 'guessology mustn't be a substitute for scientific evidence. You mustn't create recommendations out of your imagination.' Should we as a nation eat more fibre, from cereal, and vegetable, sources? 'Yet again, here is the flavour of the month,' said Dr Robertson. 'I can't go along with the "go ahead because it won't do any harm" thesis.'

This is not to suggest that Dr Robertson or any other BNF representatives expressed anything but their honestly held opinions. But it stands to reason, again, that people who work for industry or who are paid by industry are not likely to have views in conflict with the interests of industry.

In the spring of 1983 the NACNE committee had reached a predictable impasse. Wealth and health had collided. For the underlying problem, implicit in the global consensus view, is that, generally speaking, the food that is best for business is worst for health.

Added Value: for Whom?

As in other Western societies, the British food industry is a colossus, employing around two million people in growing, manufacturing, distributing and selling food. Most food eaten in Britain nowadays is highly processed. Here, for example, is the ingredients list of a packet of 'Soup in a Cup':

> Modified starch, dried glucose syrup, salt, flavour enhancers: monosodium glutamate, sodium 5-ribonucleotide; dextrose, vegetable fat, tomato powder, hydrolysed vegetable protein, yeast extract, dried oxtail, onion powder, spices, flavouring, colours: E150, E124, E102; caseinate, acidity regulator: E340; emulsifiers: E471, E472 (b); antioxidant: E320.

And here is another list of ingredients, for 'choc rolls':

> Sugar, animal and vegetable fat, flour, dextrose, whey powder, fat reduced cocoa, egg, salt, starch, skimmed milk powder, emulsifiers: E322, E435, E471; flavouring, colours: E110, E123, E142, E150.

Between them these two foods contain fats, sugars and sodium (the harmful part of salt) each in four forms, and at least 17 additives. If you look at the labels of many of the 'lead lines' in supermarkets, you will find that they are made principally of highly saturated fats, processed sugars and starches, salt, and additives.

Why? There always has been, and always will be, a clash between wealth and health, as far as food is concerned. The problem is not new. The reason is because the most profitable commodities are cheap, uniform, stable, compact, and easy to make, pack, store and transport.

Fortunes have been made from fruit and vegetables (hence 'banana republics'); but they are bulky and seasonal; they bruise, and they go bad. The qualities that make them a good food make them a bad commodity. Wholemeal flour is an unsatisfactory commodity because it goes rancid, rots, and is liable to infestation: that is to say, it supports life. Rats and weevils don't like white flour much, being sensible little chaps. By contrast, sugar is an ideal commodity: it is very stable and can be stored for years. The average consumption of processed sugars in Britain now is 100 lb a person a year, of which around 70 lb is 'hidden' in processed food. Sugars, in their various forms, are usually cheaper than the nutritious food they replace.

Food manufacturers are not trying to poison the population. The fact is, though, that good food is food that goes bad, and for much of the food industry 'shelf life' is the name of the game. Take a biscuit. The fats in a biscuit will be made from whatever is on the market, blended and 'hydrogenated'. The oils in their original state may be high in healthy polyunsaturated fatty acids or (if from palm or coconut) highly saturated and unhealthy. But the process of hydrogenation, which makes the oils into solid, stable fats, also makes them highly saturated.

This is how a biscuit on a shelf is protected against the dreaded 'seepage' and how it can carry a 'best by' date four months after you buy it. But long shelf life can lead to short human life.

'Added value' is also vital to the food industry. This means added economic value, not added value for money: value for them, not you. The more 'value' that can be added to a raw food material, the more capital can be employed and the greater the turnover. Potatoes are not much cop; the profits are in potato crisps. Wholemeal bread is not a money spinner; white bread, together with bran and germ sold as animal feed, is a better investment. An apple a day may keep the doctor away; a Mars a day helps the directors, shareholders and employees of Mars Ltd work, rest and play.

Food manufacturers therefore have a friend in the Department of Trade and Industry. The most effective firms are highly capital-intensive. For example, Kelloggs put a programme of £120 million new technology and plant investment into effect between 1983 and 1986. From 1979 to 1982 the workforce was reduced from 3,579 to 2,968, according to trade union research; and from 1979 to 1983 profits went up from £5.7 million to £41.2 million. In 1984 £28 million was spent on advertising; about the same as the total wage bill.

National and international chemical and drugs firms also have a major interest in the farming and food manufacturing industries: pesticides, herbicides, fertilizers, antibiotics, hormones and additives are all 'added value' whether the product be a loaf of bread, a joint of meat, or a chocolate roll.

By contrast, whole fresh food by definition has little or no 'added value': the value is in the food itself. Farmers raising free-range poultry, deep-sea fishermen, small master bakers, traditional cheese-makers, greengrocers and fishmongers, need plant and machinery, but their work is labour-intensive, not capital-intensive.

Such people are not, however, powerful voices in the food industry. The industry representative bodies with whom government negotiates, in private, like the Food and Drink Federation, or the Food Manufacturers Federation, are dominated by the major food manufacturers. Retailers, curiously, do not have much say when national food policy decisions are made. This is odd, because it is retailers who are best placed to know what the consumer wants.

A Public Health Scandal

The slow progress of the NACNE report through committee was much discussed in early 1983 among health professionals in the know. In 1982 Professor Geoffrey Rose, chairman of the WHO committee on heart disease, wrote in the *British Medical Journal*: 'in Britain, we are failing to prevent a preventable disease.' In 1983 Professor Rose said: 'There are no differences in principle between the NACNE recommendations and the WHO target figures.' But 'there are some in government who don't want any target figures at all.'

In America and in other countries with published and publicized dietary goals, the rates of premature death from heart disease and other diet-related diseases were dropping. Not so in Britain. Knowledgeable doctors saw this not so much as a tragedy but as a scandal. In the fifteen years between the late 1960s and the early 1980s the heart disease death rate in America had dropped by over 25 per cent. The Australian success story is similar. In British terms this would mean a saving of perhaps 40,000 lives a year. But these lives were not being saved.

One incensed doctor went as far as to say that the blocking of the NACNE report amounted to 'the biggest scandal in British public health since the Victorian days when officials refused to accept or act on the fact that cholera and typhoid are water-borne diseases.'

Copies of the later NACNE drafts had been circulated; and sometimes copied and put to use. In March 1982 the London Borough of Brent produced a working document for schools, hospitals and canteens, 'Food and Health Policy in Brent', based on a NACNE draft, that was circulated to and used by over 30 health districts.

The Doctors' Dilemma

In early 1983 *The Lancet*, the doctors' journal, had started a series of features under the general title 'Nutrition: the Changing Scene'. The medical profession has officially regarded nutrition – the study of food and health from a scientific or medical point of view – as a backwater, for the past fifty years. *The Lancet* features marked an irreversible and profound shift of British medicine, to a new recognition that good food is vital to good health.

As reflected in the national and international committee reports, knowledgeable doctors are in no doubt that fats, sugars, salt and alcohol are major public health issues. They not only replace nourishing food in the diet; there is general agreement that singly and in combination, in the quantity they are typically consumed in Western countries, they are harmful to health. Until the 1970s most research had been on fats, saturated fats in particular, and heart disease. But almost all independent scientists agree that we are all at risk from the typical British diet. The only serious dispute between independent scientists now, is just how much damage is caused by saturated fats, sugars, salt and alcohol, and just how much less we should consume.

In 1984 Sir Richard Doll was asked if he would want to change his view on food and health, as expressed in the 1982 Harveian Oration. 'I would strengthen that statement now,' he said. 'The evidence is even stronger now than it was then.'

The NACNE report also had profound implications for the medical profession. Drugs and surgery may relieve suffering from Western diseases, but such treatment does not affect the number of people who develop these diseases. And in so far as Western diseases are diet-related, the priority should be prevention, rather than treatment; in which case responsibility passes from doctors to government, industry and health educators, and of course also to the individual. But in hospitals the big money and glory is in high technology; in so far as medicine is a business, prevention is bad for business. There is no vested interest in good health.

The Revelation of NACNE

While members of the NACNE committee had not signed the Official Secrets Act they had, since 1980, treated its deliberations as strictly confidential. But word was getting out. Those concerned with public health in Britain found it difficult to answer the questions of colleagues, and to explain to foreign visitors why nothing was happening in Britain.

Geoffrey Finsberg, the minister at the DHSS then responsible for public health, addressed a private meeting of Health Education Council staff in May 1983 and, perhaps sensing restlessness, told his audience that on matters of nutrition policy the DHSS spoke for the medical consensus. He instructed the HEC to toe the DHSS line. This was confirmed a month later by Mrs Molly Disselduff, a DHSS representative on NACNE. She said in public 'there are official recommendations, and the Health Education Council follows them'. The HEC sees itself and is seen as a body of some independence, albeit funded by the DHSS, and senior HEC staff resented this instruction, which meant that their voice on NACNE must echo that of government.

On 13 June 1983 a further meeting of NACNE was held. The DHSS representative said 'we couldn't support it [the NACNE report]' as presented. Dr Derek Shrimpton, who had succeeded Dr Turner as Director-General of the BNF on 1 September 1982, said that he 'could not put his name to it'.

Nine days later, on 22 June, the BNF held its fifth annual conference, at the Royal College of Physicians. The theme of the day was 'Implementing Dietary Guidelines'. Most of the delegates were from the food industry. A number of doctors, nutritionists and people in public health had invited themselves. Professor Morris and Professor James were not present. Three of the speakers, Dr David Buss of MAFF, Mrs Disselduff of the DHSS, and Dr Juliet Gray of the BNF, were members of the main NACNE committee. No speaker throughout the day made any reference to the NACNE report.

After persistent questioning from the audience, Dr Shrimpton of the BNF acknowledged the existence of the NACNE report as a document under discussion. He then said that Professor James's sub-committee was an 'ad hoc group' and that the report would 'not be published by NACNE as such'. He said that Professor James was free to publish the report himself, if he chose.

The *Sunday Times* Report

That did it. One of the authors of this book (Geoffrey Cannon), who was then working for *The Sunday Times*, was given copies of the draft NACNE reports and published a series of reports, the first one of which was the front-page lead news story under the heading 'Censored – a Diet for Life and Death'. As a result, television, radio, magazines and other newspapers became interested in the NACNE report. This interest was shared by the editor of *The Lancet* who decided to publish much of the report in the form of four long extracts. A leader in *The Lancet* in August said that the food industry 'apparently disliked much of what it read and seems to have got the Department of Health to suppress or at any rate delay the report. If so, the Department should think again.'

The Sunday Times published a number of letters. One from Alistair Mackie, who had been Director-General of the HEC in the 1970s, read:

The suppressions and evasions of complaisant ministers, a supine Department of Health and powerful lobbyists are winning the day; and the food industry seems set to continue what a Reith lecturer called its enormous success in ruining our diet and consequently our health.

Dr Richard Turner, a signatory of a 1976 report on heart disease prevention for which the Royal College of Physicians was jointly responsible, wrote:

> In Britain the lead is never likely to come from the DHSS. As in the USA it must come from doctors and scientists whose sole interest is the health of the nation and the prevention of diet-related diseases; and from a well-informed public, not confused by commercial propaganda, or manipulation of prices by inappropriate subsidies to food producers, or misled by inadequate food labelling.

Tim Fortescue, a former Conservative MP who was at the time the boss of NACNE committee member John Wood, as Secretary-General of the Food and Drinks Industries Council, also wrote to *The Sunday Times*, contradicting Mr Mackie. Asked about the NACNE sub-committee, he said 'you mean, that little group of acolytes that James assembled around him to write his report?' and 'I don't think I have a view about dietary guidelines. They could range from the extremely stupid to the extremely sensible.' As an example of a sensible guideline, he instanced 'there should be less strychnine in food.'

From NACNE to JACNE

Professor Morris and Professor James were now in a difficult position. Interviewed, Morris said: 'Some people in the food industry are against any kind of change. Their attitude is flying in the face of an extraordinary strength of medical and scientific opinion.'

Minds concentrated by publicity, the main NACNE committee agreed to issue the report on 5 September 1983, and the HEC was asked to print it and make it available to health professionals on request. It was given the title *A Discussion*

Paper on Proposals for Nutritional Guidelines for Health Education in Britain and was sub-titled 'Prepared for the National Advisory Committee on Nutrition Education by an *ad hoc* working party under the Chairmanship of Professor W. P. T. James'. This was not the title of a report designed to enflame the public imagination, or as a crash programme for change.

Since 1983, government has been careful to distance itself fron NACNE. On 10 April 1984 Michael Meadowcroft, Liberal health spokesman, asked what was being done to implement NACNE. In reply John Patten, who had succeeded Mr Finsberg as government junior health minister, said that it was not an official report but had been issued 'to individuals and other bodies concerned with nutrition and health education, and we welcome it as a contribution to discussion.'

In the same month the *British Medical Journal* called on government 'to recognize the need for urgent action' to incorporate the reasoning of the NACNE report into its official thinking.

Two months later NACNE was disbanded, and replaced by a new committee, JACNE (short for Joint Advisory Committee on Nutrition Education) with a new chairman, Dr John Garrow. JACNE's remit included the translation of government advisory committee reports into everyday language. This did not include the NACNE report.

In December 1984 Dr Derek Shrimpton resigned as Director-General of the BNF. He had been under pressure for some time. A confidential letter written by an official of the Food Manufacturers Federation in June 1984 explained why. 'There needs to be a clearer understanding than exists now, on how far the BNF – meaning effectively its Director-General Dr Derek Shrimpton – accepts that it has a responsibility, not necessarily to "speak for the industry" (which might cause it to forfeit its credibility) but to put forward contrary views to those of cranks like the authors of *The Food Scandal*.'

Thunder and Enlightenment

By this time NACNE had been described by one London-based Professor of Nutrition as 'our own Watergate', and food and health became, in 1984, a favourite topic of conversation. The NACNE report itself is, however, written in medical language, and not designed for the general public, so media coverage tended to focus on whether or not the Department of Health and the food manufacturers' representatives on the NACNE committee had been up to no good, rather than on what Professor James and its sub-committee, and the other expert reports synthesized by NACNE, were trying to put across.

Accordingly, *The Food Scandal* was written and, on publication, was accompanied by a series of three page-long features in *The Times* (written by Geoffrey Cannon) on medical, political and commercial aspects of NACNE, together with a guide to healthy eating. These appeared on 11–13 June 1984.

Three weeks later, on 5 July 1984, Michael Jopling, the minister at MAFF, issued a press release commenting on 'the suggestions that have been made in recent weeks in the press and elsewhere that there has been some sort of conspiracy amongst food producers and processors to suppress information about the effects of diet upon health.' A week later another press release from Mr Jopling commented on 'the extremists who want to make our traditional eating habits into some kind of political scandal.'

In the meantime, *The Times* had set some kind of record by printing 30 letters in response to the three features, which had appeared under the general heading 'The Food Scandal'. Some readers were worried about food additives and contaminants. Others resented an attack on their bacon and eggs. Others said that everybody dies. Food industry representatives and their advisors (some writing from private addresses) denied that there was an established link between diet and disease. Mothers were furious about the low quality of school meals.

The President of the Royal College of Physicians said that 'there are different views about the relationship of diet to health', and that many of the links proposed between the Western diet and Western diseases remained to be proved. In reply, Professor Morris and Professor Thomas McKeown demurred. Professor McKeown, an advisor on the prevention of disease to the World Health Organization, wrote

> It is . . . often necessary to advise action on evidence which is less than complete, having regard for what has been called a 'burden of prudence' rather than a burden of proof.

Mrs Jean Waulby wrote to say that the hedgehogs in her garden were taking to their new diet of wholemeal bread. Lieutenant-Colonel Michael Moody of the Ministry of Defence spotted a lady feeding wholemeal bread to ducks in St James's Park. 'Is this the ultimate in wildlife preservation?' he asked. Commander R. J. Bassett, RAN (Retd) wrote to say that in his part of Shropshire 'wood pigeons, rooks, jackdaws, crows and doves obstinately refuse to eat the best stone-ground oven-baked bread and prefer instead the steam-processed white blotting paper.'

Food and health had indeed become part of the fabric of national debate.

About 'The Food Scandal'

The NACNE report is the only expert report published in Britain that incorporates modern medical and scientific thinking not just about one disease (like heart disease, for example) or one part of our diet (like fats), but about the British diet as a whole, and the effect of diet *as a whole* on health. It is, however, written in medical language.

So Part 1 of this book, 'The NACNE report in Everyday Language' is just that: a 'translation' of the report for the lay reader, as well as for everybody with a professional interest in the quality of food and the relationship between food, health and disease. It is what used to be called 'a plain man's guide'. Readers with special interest are encouraged also to obtain and read the chief sources of the report, listed on page 41. (An additional report, *Diet, Nutrition and Cancer*, was published by the National Research Council in the USA in 1982, by the National Academy Press: ask for it in your library.)

In Part 1, passages in the NACNE report that assume medical knowledge have been supplemented with a sentence or two of explanation, and some background information omitted from the final, published draft has been included. Some other passages not of central relevance to the report's main themes have been summarized. Some corrections have been made.

Part 2, 'Questions and Answers about Food and Health' is greatly enlarged since the first hardback edition of this book, and is concerned with themes arising from NACNE. As the title of this section of the book suggests, it answers thirty of the questions that have been debated recently, about food and health.

Part 3, 'Your Food and Your Health: What to Do', is designed as a practical guide to healthy food, for use by everybody who buys, prepares and cooks food, at home for themselves and their families, or professionally. This section of the book is also greatly enlarged and up-dated, and includes the latest information about food labelling, standards and composition. The chapters on fats and oils, meat and poultry, fish, vegetables and alcohol are rewritten and include the latest information up to April 1985.

On a point of style: this edition generally uses the terms 'fats' and 'sugars' rather than 'fat' and 'sugar'. This is because there are many different types of fats and sugars. In the case of fats, it is commonly supposed that all fats are bad for health. Happily, this is not true. Some fats are positively good for health. It is therefore best to indicate that fats are not basically one thing, at the expense of occasional clumsy phrasing. In the case of sugars, it is commonly supposed that sugar and sucrose (as in table sugar) are the same thing. This is not true. Sucrose is the commonest of a large number of sugars, all, in processed form, bad for health. So the accurate term 'sugars' is used. ('Fibre' refers to six different substances, and 'protein' is made up of a large number of amino acids, but the singular terms 'fibre' and 'protein' are used here.)

The NACNE report includes 'short-term' and also 'long-term' goals. This has confused many people. Many readers of the report have wondered which goals to go for. The answer is that the short-term goals do not represent a healthy diet; they represent simple adjustments to eating habits, such as cutting out sugars and salt at table. For health, the 'long-term' goals are the ones to go for: and you as an individual can probably reach them as from today, or at least after your next shopping expedition. Anybody who has become accustomed to eating highly processed food will be astonished to find just how delicious whole fresh food is.

Every chapter in Part 3 includes a summary of recommendations, and the book ends with an overall summary, and an example of a healthy weekly shopping basket for a family of four.

Good appetite! And long life!

PART I

The NACNE Report in Everyday Language

Food should be enjoyable, and eating and drinking is important in the family and in society. The recommendations of this report are designed to encourage a more nutritious national diet. Good and nutritious food is the most important means of preserving health and preventing disease.

The recommendations for changes in the national diet are presented as numerical goals to make planning effective; short-term as well as long-term goals are included.

The changes recommended are for the whole population. They are not only for 'vulnerable' or 'at risk' groups, such as people with high blood pressure or who suffer from heart problems or intestinal disorders, but for everybody.

The recommendations are also for people of all ages, although some additional recommendations are made for special groups: babies, young children, adolescents, the elderly and ethnic minorities.

1. THE BRITISH DIET IS UNBALANCED

For many years the concept of a 'balanced diet' has been central to nutrition education. It is said that, to ensure health, a diet should be 'balanced'.

As a principle, 'balance' is of course fine. But as applied to the food we eat, the idea is used in a special sense. It derives from the fact that the body needs a minimum amount of energy, protein, essential fats, vitamins and minerals, and that below these minimum amounts deficiency diseases develop. (Examples of these are scurvy, because of lack of vitamin C; stunted growth, because of lack of protein or energy, or both.)

Some foods – wholegrain cereals, for example – are rich in many nutrients. Other foods are rich in some nutrients, emptied of others. Thus the concept of a balanced and varied diet is that the best safeguard against deficiency diseases is to eat a large number of different foods, so that any nourishment lacking in one will be made up by another.

The 'balanced and varied' diet was designed to prevent deficiency diseases, and it was promoted most vigorously during and after the Second World War. Although it was intended to produce good health, it was not developed with the idea of preventing disorders of middle age. The importance of diet in this respect was not well recognized. The 'balanced diet' promoted during and after the war came to be regarded as 'normal', even 'perfect' for maintaining optimum health.

Nutritional deficiency diseases are no longer seen as a major public health problem in Britain or other Western societies. Instead, a number of other types of diet-related diseases have become increasingly common during this century; these are the disorders that cause premature illness and death. Heart disease is the single most common cause of premature death in the UK, as well as of deaths over the age of sixty-five.*

The 'balanced and varied' diet pays no attention to the problems caused by consumption of excessive fats, sugar and

---

*A report by Professor John Catford published in the *British Medical Journal* in December 1984 revealed that the rates of premature deaths from heart disease and strokes, respiratory diseases, all cancers, and all causes, is now higher in the UK than any other European country. Premature death rates are highest of all in Scotland and Northern Ireland.

salt, and inadequate fibre, and is out of date. Also, the notion that the average British diet is 'normal' or 'ideal' must also be abandoned, as it has been in many other Western countries where similar food is eaten. 'Balance' between foods high and low in nourishment, or between healthy foods and those that cause disease, is a false idea of balance.

For these reasons, the term 'prudent diet' has become popular in the United States. This is the term for a healthy diet which prevents both deficiency diseases and diseases of middle age. However, because the term 'prudent' seems to imply restriction and discipline, a better term is 'healthy diet'.

Together with 'balanced and varied' diet, other terms still used in nutrition education should be discarded. In particular, foods are still grouped as 'protein foods' (good for growth and body repair); 'energy foods' (for use in work); and 'protective foods' (especially rich in vitamins and minerals). Here again, the idea has been one of 'balance'. A food such as sugar which is heavy in calories but empty of protein, vitamins and minerals has been regarded as acceptable because it could be 'balanced' by other nutritious foods.

Such a grouping is now inappropriate for many reasons. One is that it encourages the idea that processed fats and sugars are valuable foods, whereas many other foods contain not only calories but also protein, vitamins and minerals. Another is that it leads to arbitrary and misleading classification: many types of meat and dairy produce, together with milk, should, for example, be seen as high-fat foods, rather than (as they now are) 'protein foods'.

A Policy For the Nation as a Whole

Different people eat different foods. A recent survey in Cambridgeshire showed that the average intake of dietary fibre was about ¾ oz (20 grams) a day and of fat about 3½ oz (100 grams) a day. But fibre intake ranged from 8 to 32 grams a day and fat from 20 to 170 grams a day.

Given that the population as a whole should eat more fibre and less fat, this variation suggests that the best nutrition policy might be to concentrate on those people who eat remarkably little fibre, or remarkably large amounts of fat – or both.

But the detection of people with extreme habits would be extraordinarily time-consuming and difficult. In any case, individuals are more or less susceptible (or 'sensitive' or 'vulnerable') to different foods, so that a high intake of fat may be harmful to one person but not to another.

For example, it is well established that too much saturated fat in the diet (as in the typical British diet) is harmful and is a basic cause of heart disease. If we could find all the people who eat most saturated fat, and if they then changed their eating habits, would it solve the problem of heart disease in Britain? Unfortunately it would not. The reason is that the people who develop heart disease are not only those whose intake of saturated fat is especially high. Very large numbers of them consume about the average amount of saturated fat; they are at the 'middling' level. Some are even people who, although they eat rather little saturated fat compared with most others, are unusually sensitive to it. The problem is that the majority of us in Britain have a high level of saturated fat in our food. Only if the population as a whole reduces the quantity eaten will the problem of heart disease be dealt with effectively.

Cholesterol is another similar problem. A high level of cholesterol in the blood is an established cause of heart disease. The higher the level, the higher the risk of having a premature heart attack. (High blood cholesterol is itself caused by high levels of saturated fat and cholesterol in food, aggravated by cigarette smoking and lack of exercise.) An examination of levels of blood cholesterol shows that a few people have a very high level, a few a very low level, but that the vast majority have 'middling' levels, around the average. This is the case in all countries where blood cholesterol has been measured in large numbers of people. The UK, together with other Western countries, stands out because the population as a whole has such a high blood cholesterol level. It might be thought that, if only we could locate people with a very high level (by giving them a blood test), the problem of heart disease would be solved because such people could then be given appropriate advice and/or treatment. However, even in the UK there are very few such people: about five in every hundred. So, although the risk to their health as individuals is very great (their chance of having a premature heart attack might be two or three times that of someone with a low blood cholesterol level), the actual number of deaths each year among such individuals is relatively very small. There are too few of them to make a big difference to the death figures.

By far the largest number of deaths (about 90 per cent) occurs among the enormous number of people whose blood cholesterol is around the 'middling' or average level, simply because the average level in the UK is so high. Their individual risk is lower than those with very high blood cholesterol, but because there are so many of them, the public health problem they cause is very large.

The point about all this is that, first of all, you cannot predict which level of blood cholesterol will be particularly harmful to you personally – individuals are different. By the time you know that you have reached your limit, it may well be too late; disease will have developed already and more likely than not, there will have been no warning symptoms. Second, we know that the 'middling' level of blood cholesterol in Britain is very high by world standards. It is the enormous number of people with 'middling' levels who cause the public health problem. The sensible and logical approach, therefore, is for all of us to eat a healthy diet and prevent our blood cholesterol going up in the first place. Prevention is better than cure. And in the case of heart attacks, many deaths are so sudden that treatment is out of the question.

The best policy, therefore, is not to concentrate on groups within the population whose eating habits are unusual, but, instead, to emphasize the benefits to everybody of changes in the national diet. Our present national diet is unhealthy; all of us are at risk of premature illness as a result.

So, everybody should eat less fat. Likewise, everybody should eat more dietary fibre, and less sugar and salt. Here, the same sorts of arguments apply. The less dietary fibre eaten, the greater the risk of various bowel disorders. And the more salt eaten, the greater the risk of high blood pressure and therefore of heart disease. But sufferers from bowel disorders and high blood pressure do not eat remarkably low amounts of fibre or remarkably high amounts of salt, compared with the UK national average.

Again, this is because individuals' susceptibility to lack of fibre and too much salt varies. It is also because the British national average intake of fibre is unhealthy, being too low, and the average intake of salt is unhealthy, being too high – as is that of fats and sugars.

It has been established for some years that the British diet is unhealthy. But, until now, recommendations for change have been vague and have not provided those professionally concerned with food and health with a clear set of goals.

In this report, figures are given for recommended average intakes of fibre, fat, sugar and salt; and percentage figures are given for recommended changes from current average intakes. In addition, short-term goals are given (for the 1980s) and also long-term goals (for the 1980s and 1990s).

Recommendation

- The recommendations of the report are for the population as a whole, not for 'at risk' groups. The typical British diet puts us all at risk.
- The recommendations are for average intake for the population, and not for each individual person.

2. OVERWEIGHT: NEED FOR NEW ADVICE

Overweight is very common in Britain. More than half of all men and four out of ten women over the age of forty are overweight. The problem is not confined to middle age: in the sixteen- to nineteen-year-old age group, three out of twenty are overweight. The figures for adults of all ages are, on average, 39 per cent of men and 32 per cent of women i.e. more than one-third of all adults in Britain are overweight.

The figures for obese people, those who are so overweight that they run immediate risks to their health, are of course lower. Of all adults in Britain, 6 per cent of men and 8 per cent of women are obese.

Mild Overweight Is Dangerous

Obese people are liable to have health problems, and they run a higher risk of suffering and dying from various diseases. The risks to health increase as the degree of overweight increases.

But it is also true that people who are only slightly overweight, rather than obese, run risks with their health. This is especially the case with people who have a family history of heart disease or diabetes, or who themselves have high blood pressure.

Overweight in the Family

Four diseases that overweight people are more likely to suffer from are heart disease, high blood pressure, diabetes and gall bladder disease. Together with heart disease, high blood pressure and diabetes, obesity is liable to 'run in the family'. These are conditions that tend to recur in the children – and the grandchildren – of sufferers.

It is especially important that people in such families do not gain weight in adult life and do not become overweight.

At the same time, a substantial proportion of the population becomes overweight, and so more liable to disease, without having a family history of overweight or disease. On average the British people are gradually becoming more overweight. Moreover, overweight children and young adults are very likely to remain overweight or become obese in later life.

Smoking and Bodyweight

Smoking is more dangerous than overweight. Even though smokers weigh less than non-smokers, their risk of developing premature disease is greater.

Smoking speeds up the metabolic rate. When people give up smoking they are liable to gain weight, partly because their metabolic rate goes down, and partly because their appetite tends to increase.

People who give up smoking should eat less, or exercise more, to avoid weight gain. On a long-term basis, ex-smokers should change their diet. In particular, they should cut down their consumption of fat and sugar.

Different People, Different Needs

Fat people are not characteristically greedy. While it is true that some people become fat because of eating great quantities of food, this is not usually the reason why people get fat. Two people may be the same weight, height, shape and appearance, and yet need remarkably different amounts of food. One such person may stay the same weight, while the other – eating no more food – will gain weight. Overweight children and adults will often have to be very diligent and careful if they are to lose weight, or avoid gaining more weight.

Slimming and Exercise

People who want to lose weight and to maintain their weight loss should realize that the advice given up to now on weight loss and weight control has often been wrong.

First, the rapid weight loss that results from popular diet regimes consists principally not of lost fat but of water, together with glycogen (the body's immediately available store of energy) and lean body tissue.

To be effective, weight loss should be at the rate of one to two pounds a week and no more. It follows that many overweight people will need several months to lose their excess weight effectively.

Second, the advice that, in order to lose weight, the diet should simply contain less of every common food, is wrong. People in Britain and other Western countries eat too many fats and sugars. Much of this is 'hidden' in meat and meat products, in the case of fats, and in most processed foods, in the case of sugars. At the volume they are eaten in Britain, fats and sugars are bad for health and are also a prime cause of overweight. Effective weight loss and the maintenance of target weight requires a permanent reduction of fats and sugars.

The pattern of food eaten, and the choice of foods, is important. In place of fat and sugar, healthy choices are more cereals, bread, vegetables and fruit.

Everybody should be encouraged to take regular, vigorous exercise throughout life. In particular, overweight and middle-aged people should be encouraged to be more active. There is evidence that people who eat small amounts of food, but who are relatively inactive, are more likely to suffer and die from heart disease. More facilities for exercise are needed in the community, including at places of work.

Sugars and Overweight

Whole foods are best for weight loss and also for maintaining normal weight. Whole foods may be quite high in energy; but because they are bulky as well as nourishing, they are satisfying.

Sugars contain calories but no nourishment. Because of the

refining process they are also a very concentrated source of calories. Sugars tend to 'fool' the body into consuming an unnecessary amount of energy. Studies have shown that when an artificial sweetening agent free of calories replaces sugars in the diet, people consume the same volume of food and therefore less energy. This is true for both overweight and normal weight people.*

It follows that any concentrated processed food is liable to cause overweight.

So many people in Britain are overweight, or liable to become overweight, that the only sensible approach is a change in everybody's eating habits. A fundamental change in certain current attitudes to foods is also needed.

National consumption of fats should be reduced by a quarter, and of sugars by half. Apart from energy, fats contain little nourishment, and sugars contain no nourishment. So cutting down the amount of fats and sugars eaten reduces the amount of calories consumed without reducing the intake of essential nutrients – for example, protein, vitamins and minerals.

A permanent national reduction in fats and sugars would do a great deal to prevent overweight children becoming overweight, and possibly obese, adults.

Carbohydrates are commonly supposed to be fattening foods. This is an error. It is vital that those concerned with health education, and the public in general, realize that foods containing large amounts of carbohydrate as starch (such as bread and potatoes) are not in themselves fattening.

---

*In a key experiment published in 1983, Dr Kenneth Heaton and co-workers gave two diets to volunteers. The volunteers were asked to eat until they were satisfied. The average calorie intake of the low-sugar eaters was 1700; of the high-sugar eaters 2180 – over 25 per cent more. Heaton proposed that 'energy intake is unwittingly inflated when refined carbohydrate foods are consumed'.

Recommendation

- Overweight people should not usually eat less, but exercise more. At the same time, they should change their eating patterns.

3. SUGARS, OBESITY AND TOOTH DECAY

For decades, people have been told that the right way to lose weight is to eat less of all carbohydrates. This advice is wrong for slimmers, and wrong for the population as a whole. Everybody should be told that such advice is wrong.

Obese people may well react to food in a different way from people of normal weight. In particular, obese people tend not to burn dietary fat but to store it as body fat instead, to a greater extent than people of normal weight. Overweight people should therefore cut down on fats and substitute carbohydrate-rich foods for fatty foods.

But a sharp distinction should be drawn between different types of carbohydrate. Starches and sugars are both carbohydrate: both supply energy to the body. Whole foods rich in starch, such as wholemeal bread, potatoes and other cereals and vegetables, are nutritious and also rich in fibre. On average, the recommendation is that we eat half as much again of these foods.

On the other hand, refined sugars, have no nutritional value, and certainly contribute to obesity. The recommendation here, is to eat half as much sugar as we now eat.

The advice to eat less fats, less sugars and more whole food rich in fibre applies equally to people who need to lose weight, to people at risk of diseases, and to the whole population.

Sugars and Tooth Decay

Sugars are the primary cause of tooth decay. Throughout the world it has been demonstrated that the more sugars people eat, the more their teeth rot. As examples, people in China and Ethiopia eat very little sugars and have excellent teeth. In Japan and Hungary rather more sugars are eaten and the rate of tooth decay is rather higher.

In Britain we eat on average about 4½ oz (125 grams) of sugars a day, or about 100 lb (45·4 kg) a year*. By the age of eleven or twelve, British children have on average over eight decayed, missing or filled teeth.

The bacteria involved in tooth decay do not do their work without the presence of sugars or some comparable processed foods. Fluoridation of the water supply and of toothpaste, and regular brushing of teeth, reduces tooth decay but does not prevent it.

Sugars come in different forms, including sucrose, glucose, dextrose, fructose and maltose. These all rot teeth. Sticky sweet food, and sweet food eaten as snacks or drunk between meals, is extremely damaging to teeth.

All this is hotly disputed by the sugar industry and their paid representatives. By contrast, some medical and dental authorities recommend dramatic cuts in sugar consumption, to 25-40 lb a year. One British authority states that, given fluoridation, an upper limit of 32 lb a year should prove safe as far as tooth decay is concerned.

The foods to cut down most of all are sweets, other confectionery, soft drinks and sweet snacks. The recommended

---

*There is an error in the NACNE report. At one point it cites correctly a Ministry of Agriculture figure that the average sucrose consumption in Britain is 83½ lb (38 kg) a year. But at another point in the report this figure is confused with total sugars consumption (a common error). The 1982 figures (much the same as 1980) show that when the figures for consumption of glucose, dextrose, fructose and sugars used to make alcoholic drinks are added to sucrose consumption, the total average British sugar consumption is 101.6 lb (46.2 kg) a year. In round figures, the British eat on average 100 lb of sugars a year. It follows that the NACNE recommendation that we halve consumption of sugars (to 50 lb a year) is slightly at odds with the upper recommended limit of 44 lb (20 kg) a year. From the point of view of good health, the upper limit of 44 lb should stand.

upper limit of such foods is 1 oz a day, which amounts to 22 lb (10 kg) a year. Sugar contained in foods eaten as meals is less damaging to teeth, and the recommended upper limit is also 22 lb a year. Thus the total recommended upper limit of all forms of refined sugars is 44 lb (20 kg) a year.

If sugars in the form of soft drinks and snacks are reduced still further, so much the better. From all points of view, it is easier to cut down sugar in this relatively obvious form than in processed foods eaten at meals. But overweight people are best advised to avoid refined sugars in all forms.

Recommendation

- Sugars: consumption should be cut by one half or thereabouts, to 10 per cent of total calorie intake from the present level of 20 per cent.
- Sugars in snacks: consumption should be no more than half the total intake of sugars, or five per cent of total calorie intake.

4. FIBRE: PROTECTS GOOD HEALTH

Lack of fibre causes constipation. We are a constipated nation. Two out of every five people in Britain say that they are constipated. Nearly four out of five people pass only five to seven stools each week. One in ten people pass three or four stools or even less. Almost one in five British people take laxatives. British people eat little fibre. Currently on average we consume about ¾ oz (20 grams) a day. During the war, when British people ate bread made from brown flour with more fibre in it, and more potatoes, fibre consumption was 1 to 1½ oz (32 to 40 grams) a day. Vegetarians in the UK consume over twice the national average of fibre – 1½ oz (42 grams) a day.

Low intakes of fibre are associated with various disorders of the gut; not only constipation, but also the irritable bowel syndrome, diverticular disease, and cancer of the colon. Diverticular disease (the development of little pockets in the intestinal wall which can become inflamed) is very common, affecting one in five of people in the West aged fifty to sixty, and two in five of those between sixty and seventy. Cancer of the large bowel is the second most common cancer in Britain, killing one in eight of all people who die of cancer in England and Wales (1980 figures). Evidence of the link between lack of fibre and disorders of the gut was initially obtained by comparing Western societies and rural communities in the Third World. Africans living away from Western influence eat 2 to 4½ oz of fibre (55 to 125 grams) a day. Constipation, together with various disorders of the gut, is rare or unknown in these communities. Diverticular disease is also less common among vegetarians. This evidence now has firm experimental and clinical backing.

It is thought that by increasing the bulk of stools and speeding up the flow through the lower gut and the bowel, fibre exercises the intestines, reduces pressure, prevents straining at stool, and dilutes the waste matters in stools that are potential causes of cancer. Lack of fibre produces small, hard, abrasive stools with a concentrated toxic content.

Cereal fibre eaten in the form of whole grains (wholemeal bread, for example, or muesli) has a more marked effect on the bulk of stools than the vegetable or fruit fibres so far studied.

How Much More Fibre Should We Eat?

The recommendation is that on average we should eat half as much fibre again. Intake should increase to just over 1 oz (30 grams) a day. This increase will certainly go a long way to reduce constipation and diverticular disease.

Cereal foods are the most effective source of fibre so far studied, from the point of view of increasing the weight and volume of stools, and speeding up their passage through the intestines. Everybody would also be advised to eat more fruit and vegetables. (Much of the medical research on fibre has concentrated on wheat fibre–bran–in the context of a Western diet; less work has been done on the effects of typically 'non-Western' foods such as brown and white rice and pasta, beans and tropical vegetables. Such foods undoubtedly are helpful to the digestive process but less is known about them.)

The best source of fibre is whole food. Much attention is paid nowadays to special 'high fibre' preparations in the form of tablets; or to foods to which fibre, usually in the form of bran, has been added; or to bran for sprinkling on foods or for use in cooking. These fibre 'supplements' are not the best form of fibre. Whole food should always be preferred. There is evidence that bran, and perhaps other foods also high in fibre, may to some extent deprive the body of some minerals. Any such effect is more than compensated for by eating mineral-rich whole food.

Recommendation

- Fibre: consumption should be increased by one half, to 30 grams a day, from the present level of 20 grams a day. This should take the form of whole food: cereals, and also vegetables and fruit.

5. FATS, CHOLESTEROL, HEART DISEASE

Fat in food is a major cause of heart disease. This is not seriously disputed by the expert committees in Britain and elsewhere concerned with the prevention of heart disease. The question is, rather, which types of fat are particularly harmful, and what is the amount by which we should reduce our consumption of fats.

Heart disease is the biggest single killer in Britain. Northern Ireland and Scotland (with Finland) have the highest rate of death from heart disease in the world, and England and Wales are not far behind.

Heart disease is also a major cause of premature death. In 1980, 31 per cent – nearly one third – of all deaths from heart disease in England and Wales were in men under the age of sixty-five.

Worse, while in recent years the death rate from heart disease has been dropping in many countries, including the USA, Canada, Australia, Belgium, the Netherlands and Finland, there has been no significant fall in the UK.

In Britain we eat on average about 4½ oz (125 g) of fats a day, or about 100 lb (45·4 kg) a year: roughly the same weight as sugars. But because fats are much heavier in calories than sugars, they provide a large amount (about 38 per cent) of our total calorie intake. (The 38 per cent figure includes calories from alcohol; if alcohol is excluded, as it is in some calculations, the figure for fats is 40–41 per cent of calories.)

Some expert committees recommend a drop in the percentage of calories from fats to 30 per cent, others to 35 per cent. (The difference may partly be explained by including or excluding calories from alcohol.)

A key way of reducing the risk of heart disease is to lower the level of cholesterol in the blood. It is reliably estimated that in order to bring down cholesterol in the blood to a reasonably safe level, the target for calories from fats should be 30 per cent of total energy intake. The benefits of limiting the intake of saturated fats and total fats by people with high levels of cholesterol in the blood are established.

Blood cholesterol levels can be brought down even lower by limiting calories from fats to below 30 per cent of total energy. This level of fats consumption is still well in excess of that found in the Third World where blood cholesterol is also much lower. Further reductions of fat intake, stringent for people accustomed to Western food, might not in any case reduce the risk of heart disease further for adults. For children, the lower the fat intake the better.

Saturated Fats and Heart Disease

Saturated fats, which lead to blockages in the arteries, are a major underlying cause of heart disease. About half the fats we eat are in the form of saturated fats. Most saturated fats are solid in form and of animal origin; exceptions are coconut oil and palm oil, much used in food processing, and also processed vegetable oils.

There is general agreement that there should be a big reduction in intake of saturated fats.

The recommendation is that we should reduce our intake of saturated fats by about half, from 18 per cent of total energy intake to 10 per cent.

Polyunsaturated Fats: Protective?

Polyunsaturated fats are not a cause of heart disease. Rather, they may have a protective role. We eat only small amounts of polyunsaturated fats: about 4 per cent of total energy intake. Most polyunsaturated fats are liquid in their natural form (oils) and are of vegetable and fish origin.

Expert committees have different views about polyunsaturated fats. Most propose a positive increase in consumption, as a protective measure. There is, however, some evidence that, while reducing the rate of death from heart disease, such a policy, if it resulted in increased consumption of processed polyunsaturates rather than fats from whole food, might increase the rate of death from some cancers.

The clear and vital message about fats is: eat less saturated fats. In practice, if the target of 10 per cent of total calories from saturated fats is achieved, the amount of polyunsaturated fats eaten relative to saturated fats will increase. No doubt many people will substitute oils high in polyunsaturates for solid fats. Meat and dairy produce (both very high in saturated fats) make up about 55 per cent of our total consumption of fats. (The figures are about 30 per cent from dairy produce and 27 per cent from meat.) These are the types of fat we should cut down substantially. Instead, we should eat more cereal foods and fish, beans and other vegetables, all good sources of polyunsaturated fats. If food manufacturers chose to cut down the saturated fats used to make food and to use polyunsaturates instead, this would do no harm.

The need to reduce total fat consumption, and saturated fat in particular, should be emphasized. (A small increase in intake of polyunsaturated fat by 3 or 4 grams a day, or around 1 per cent of total calorie intake, would not do harm. In addition, given the saturated fat target, it would substantially change the ratio of the two types of fat consumed, from 9:2 to 4:2. Intake of polyunsaturated fats would therefore rise from two ninths to one half of saturated fats intake.)*

---

*The NACNE report fails to make a clear statement about polyunsaturated fats; likewise, the subsequent report, *Diet and Cardiovascular Disease* (July 1984) from the Committee on Medical Aspects on Food Policy (COMA). The basic message of NACNE, that consumption of all fats should be cut from 40 to 30 per cent of total calories, and consumption of saturated fats should be cut sharply from 18 to 10 per cent of total calories, follows the broad international scientific consensus. But what about polyunsaturated, and come to that monounsaturated, fats? The American McGovern report recommends equal consumption of all three main types of fats: saturated 10, monounsaturated 10, polyunsaturated 10 per cent of total calories. Should we consume more than the current level of 4 per cent of total calories from polyunsaturates? NACNE and COMA skate round the issue.

This is because some studies have shown that consuming an artificially high level of polyunsaturated fats can increase the risk of cancer. Previously it was supposed, over-enthusiastically, that polyunsaturates promoted health in all circumstances, and millions of Americans got into the habit of consuming great quantities of margarines almost as if they were medicine. Hence the muted NACNE message about polyunsaturates.

In practice, consuming less visible fats and oils in general, but also switching from butter to margarine marked 'high in polyunsaturates', together with consuming more whole food rich in polyunsaturates, will result in a diet with a healthy 7–10 per cent of calories supplied by polyunsaturated fats.

Cholesterol in Food, and Heart Disease

It is not clear to what extent cholesterol eaten as food raises the level of cholesterol in the blood. Scientists disagree on this point.

Some expert committees do recommend eating less cholesterol; eggs, notably. But the recommendations made in this report will have the effect of reducing dietary cholesterol and, more important, cholesterol in the blood; therefore no specific recommendation about dietary cholesterol is made here.

Other links between food and heart disease have been made. For example, there may be a link between lack of fibre, or else lack of the mineral selenium, and heart disease.

Links between non-dietary factors and heart disease – for example, smoking and lack of exercise – have already been mentioned.

Exercise and Heart Disease

Regular vigorous exercise reduces the risk of heart disease. By contrast, as already stated, people who eat small amounts of food and who are physically inactive are more likely to suffer from heart disease.

Indeed there is evidence that regular vigorous exercise reduces the risk of heart disease even if a person's diet is itself liable to produce heart disease (because it contains too much fat, for example).

Recommendation

- Fats: consumption should be cut by one quarter, to 30 per cent of total calorie intake from the present level of 38 per cent.
- Saturated fats: consumption should be cut by nearly one half, to 10 per cent of total calorie intake from the present level of 18 per cent.

• Polyunsaturated fats: there is no recommendation to increase the amount eaten. But the ratio of polyunsaturated to saturated fats will rise because of the cut in saturated fats.

6. SALT, HIGH BLOOD PRESSURE AND STROKES

Salt (sodium chloride) is a cause of high blood pressure, which in turn is a major risk factor for both heart disease and strokes.

Heart disease and strokes are major public health problems in Western countries. In England and Wales in 1980 the number of deaths ascribed to high blood pressure was 6,893; to heart disease 160,458; and to strokes 73,532. This totals 240,883 – virtually a quarter of a million people a year. The total of deaths from these causes under the age of sixty-five was also very high: 47,028 – nearly fifty thousand people.

In Western countries, blood pressure tends to rise with age; and the definition of what is 'high blood pressure' varies. In one study of 3,000 Scotsmen aged between forty-five and sixty-four, two fifths had blood pressure high enough to be medically defined as 'mildly high' – which means high enough to be a case for treatment. (The exact figure was 39.8 per cent; the blood pressure above 90 mmHg diastolic.) One quarter of the same group were significantly higher (above 95 mmHg diastolic). In the USA well over one in every ten people aged thirty-five to sixty-four have blood pressure high enough to need medical treatment.

In many Third World societies little touched by Western influence, high blood pressure is unknown, and blood pressure does not rise with age. Societies in transition between a traditional way of life and a Western style of life start to show high blood pressure along Western patterns. On the other hand, some societies, notably the Japanese and some regions of India, have very high rates of high blood pressure and also high rates of death from strokes.

People, and whole societies, free of high blood pressure, tend to have certain characteristics in common. They are slim, they exercise a lot, they eat small amounts of animal (saturated) fats; they eat large amounts of the mineral potassium and correspondingly low amounts of sodium.

Overweight and obesity are linked with high blood pressure, but are not its only cause. Likewise, a high consumption of fat, notably saturated fat, is linked with high blood pressure, but cannot be its main single cause. For example the Japanese eat little fat but have high blood pressure, and as fat intake increases in Japan the rate of death from strokes is falling.

There is strong experimental and clinical evidence linking salt with high blood pressure. There is also evidence that, just as different people are born with varying susceptibility to disease, a proportion, perhaps one in five, may be especially susceptible to salt.

When animals are fed very high levels of salt, their blood pressure rises. When strains of animal known to be susceptible to blood pressure are fed small extra amounts of salt, their blood pressure rises. When people are fed diets low in salt, their blood pressure drops. Also, sodium and potassium work together in the body: high levels of potassium counteract the bad effects of sodium.

Every known population in the world that eats low amounts of salt has no problem with high blood pressure. Every population that eats high amounts of salt does have a high blood pressure problem.

Eating less salt is likely to cause a modest drop in the population's average blood pressure. But even a small fall would bring as much benefit to a whole population as is now achieved by drug therapy. We should consume less salt.

How Much Less Salt Should We Consume?

The World Health Organization recommends an upper limit of 5 grams a day. (Note, this is 2 grams of sodium a day.) And the WHO report (*Prevention of Coronary Heart Disease*, published in 1982) points out that societies without high blood pressure problems usually consume under 3 grams of salt a day.

Average salt intakes in Britain are not known. The Ministry of Agriculture estimate is 8 grams a day. Other estimates are higher – 12 grams a day. These levels are two or even four times more than the WHO guideline.

In Britain we add substantial amounts of salt to food, in cooking and at table. But most of the salt we eat is 'hidden' in manufactured foods, not all of which taste especially salty. The same is true of sugars. Over two thirds of the sugars we eat are in manufactured foods. The figure for salt is higher: maybe four fifths.

There is therefore a sharp limit to what an individual can do by cutting down salt in cooking and at table.

Necessary reductions will involve the support of food manufacturers and must therefore be seen as long-term goals.

Government and industry should accept the need for clear and informative food labels with details of total fibre, fats, sugars, and salt content. People professionally concerned with food and health, together with everybody who buys and eats food, should be able to know what is in the food they eat.

Recommendation

• Salt: consumption should be cut by about one half, to 5 grams a day from the present level of 8–12 grams a day. Five grams of salt is 2 grams of sodium.

7. ALCOHOL, LIVER DISEASE AND ALCOHOLISM

Alcohol is a major cause of liver disease: notably cirrhosis of the liver. It is also associated with a large number of other disorders and diseases of the digestion, the gut, the heart and blood vessels, the lungs, the muscles, the nervous system, the blood and the immune system.

Any of these conditions may develop in drinkers who do not regard themselves, and who are not regarded by others, as alcoholic. However, alcohol is addictive for susceptible individuals, and the rate of alcoholism is increasing.

The risk of liver disease, notably cirrhosis, is much higher in drinkers than in non-drinkers; and the risk steadily rises according to how much the person drinks and for how many years. During Prohibition in the USA, the national average of alcohol drunk fell, and so did the rate of chronic liver disease.

It is not, however, possible to state for everyone an alcohol intake below which the risk of liver disease is low and above which it is high. As with fats, sugars and salt, people vary greatly in their susceptibility to alcohol.

Several studies have shown that in small amounts alcohol may help to protect against heart disease. It has this effect by increasing a beneficial type of fat in the blood (high density lipoprotein or HDL) and correspondingly decreasing the type of fat in the blood associated with high risk of heart disease (low density lipoprotein or LDL). While these studies are reliable, their findings should be treated with caution*. The protective amount of alcohol is quite small: about 20 to 25 grams a day, equivalent to 4–5 per cent of total energy intake, or 1½ pints of beer (or three small glasses of wine) a day. There is no evidence that consumption above this level is helpful. On the other hand, there is evidence that alcohol does no good and is liable to do harm in other ways, certainly with heavy drinkers.

As with sugars, because alcohol contains no nourishment,

---

*New studies published in 1984 suggest that the type ('subfraction') of high density lipoprotein increased by alcohol may well not protect against heart disease. It has been pointed out that some middle-aged male heart disease specialists are not as hard on alcohol as they might be, for personal reasons. This remains a controversial area.

the more people drink alcohol the less well nourished they are. Alcoholics who eat low-quality food are known sometimes to develop manifest deficiency diseases (such as beri-beri or scurvy, caused by gross lack of vitamin B_1 and vitamin C respectively).

Alcohol is not really a food; it provides calories but – in the form of alcoholic drinks – little or no nourishment. From the health point of view there is little to be said for alcohol.

The Cost of Drinking

Consumption of alcohol has risen steadily in the past twenty years for two associated reasons. First, people on the whole have had more money to spend. Second – significant at times of national economic depression – the real cost of alcohol has dropped. Figures for 1950 and 1980 show that the cost of bread has stayed much the same; the cost of beer has fallen by one third; and the cost of whisky has dropped precipitately, by over three quarters.

The cheaper alcohol is in relation to other goods, the more we drink.

Alcohol consumption varies in different parts of Britain. In the South East, the average consumption is 20 grams a day (4 per cent of energy intake, or 1 pint of beer a day). In Scotland, the figure is more than twice as high: 9 per cent of energy intake. The national average intake of alcohol is 6 per cent of total energy.

Alcohol and Alcoholism

Alcohol is liable to be addictive. Heavy drinking leading to alcoholism, and steady drinking increasing the risk of liver and other diseases, are separate public health problems.

In their report on alcoholism, the Royal College of Psychiatrists recommend an upper limit of 4 pints of beer (or 1 bottle of wine) a day. Measured as alcohol, this amounts to 60 grams a day or 12 per cent of total energy intake. Measured as beer or wine, with their sugars and other solids, the total for a basically sedentary person is 20 to 30 per cent of total energy intake. (The exact figure varies according to the type of drink and between men and women.)

This recommendation is designed to help avert alcoholism, not to promote health. For health, on the other hand, the recommended upper limit is no more than two drinks a day for men, and roughly no more than one drink a day for women (averaged out over a week).

Unlike the recommendations for fats, sugars and salt, which refer to the whole population, it is best to concentrate on lowering the alcohol intake of heavy drinkers, rather than recommending that everybody who drinks should drink less. This will have the effect of lowering the national average alcohol intake towards the recommended 4 per cent.

Recommendation

- Alcohol: consumption should be cut by one third, to 4 per cent of total energy intake, from the present level of 6 per cent.

8. PROTEIN: ANIMAL OR VEGETABLE?

The amount of protein eaten in Britain has not changed much throughout this century, remaining at about 11–12 per cent of total energy intake.

During this period, however, there has been a steady move away from vegetable (and cereal) foods, towards animal (meat and dairy) foods, so that the population now obtains a greater proportion of protein from animal rather than plant foods. The value of vegetable protein has until recently been downgraded by doctors and nutritionists.

There is no practical foundation for the still widely held

view that animal protein is superior to, or 'first class' compared with, vegetable protein. This is true for children as well as for adults.

Recommendation

- Protein: no change overall; but the amount of animal protein should decrease, and the amount of vegetable protein increase.

9. VITAMINS AND MINERALS

The Department of Health (DHSS) publishes lists of recommended daily amounts (RDAs) of some vitamins and minerals for different groups in the population. Some groups of people are known to be deficient in some vitamins and minerals. Four problems are discussed here.

Iron and Anaemia

Lack of iron is a cause of anaemia. Iron deficiency is fairly common in Britain. Menstruation and pregnancy increase women's need for iron.

Meat is rich in iron, but this report does not advocate an increase in meat consumption for anaemic people. Iron is added to white flour and so to white bread, but in a form that the body cannot readily absorb. What, then, should be done for people deficient in iron?

The body normally adapts to a low intake of iron by increasing the absorption of what iron is available. One of the functions of vitamin C is to increase the absorption of iron. The vitamin C in fruit (including citrus fruits) and in vegetables (including green leafy vegetables and potatoes) will enable us to make better use of the iron in food.

Women who cannot adapt to menstrual loss of blood or who

for other reasons such as pregnancy become anaemic, should take iron supplements.

Vitamin C, Cooking and the Common Cold

Gross deficiency of vitamin C causes scurvy. The DHSS recommended daily intake of vitamin C is three times as much as is reckoned to prevent scurvy; and on average people in Britain consume nearly twice the DHSS recommended amount of vitamin C.

But because much vitamin C is lost in the cooking – and especially the over-cooking – of food, and because of the variability of food buying habits, it is estimated that one in ten people in Britain consumes less vitamin C than the DHSS recommends.

The recommendation of this report, that we eat more fruit and vegetables, will increase the consumption of vitamin C.

It is popularly believed that taking very high doses of vitamin C in the form of supplements helps to prevent various disorders, notably the common cold. There is as yet no reliable evidence for this theory.

Folic Acid, Anaemia and Spina Bifida

Lack of folic acid (a B vitamin) cause a form of anaemia. There is evidence that lack of folic acid is also a cause of neural tube defects in the newborn, of which the best known to the public is spina bifida. Pregnancy increases the need for folic acid.

While there is no current DHSS recommended intake of folic acid*, there is reason to believe that folic acid deficiency

---

* Is there, or isn't there, a DHSS recommended daily intake for folic acid? In early 1985 this was a matter for conjecture. The official DHSS guide, *Recommended Daily Amounts of Food Energy and Nutrients for Groups of People in the United Kingdom* published by HMSO, was one of the sources for the NACNE report. Its 1969 edition contained no recommendation (RDA) for folic acid. But the 1979 edition did contain an RDA of 300

is common in Britain. Groups notably affected include pregnant women and their babies, the elderly and people of Asian descent.

The relationship between folic acid deficiency and neural tube defects is currently being investigated by the Medical Research Council, in a five year study started in 1984.

About one in seven people over the age of seventy shows signs of folic acid deficiency.

Like vitamin C, folic acid, together with all the B vitamins, is soluble in water and so largely lost in cooking. Milk in its natural state is a good source of folic acid, but 80 per cent is destroyed by pasteurization.

Folic acid is so called because it is often found in foliage – leafy vegetables. The recommendation of this report that we eat more vegetables will increase consumption of folic acid, vitamin C, and other vitamins and minerals.

Women planning a child should ensure that their diet contains plenty of green leafy vegetables, and possibly take folic acid supplements (in the form of a B complex supplement with adequate B_6, B_{12} and folic acid levels, together with zinc). The time to take such supplements is before conception.

Calcium and Children

Calcium helps children to grow. Free supplies of milk to

micrograms (mcg) a day. However, in the 1981 edition (cited in the NACNE report) the 1979 recommendation had disappeared.

The plot then thickened. The Ministry of Agriculture, Fisheries and Food (MAFF), the other government department with an interest, as from 19 September 1984 has allowed food manufacturers to make claims on food labels for the folic acid content of foods, relative to a recommended daily intake of 300 mcg. This is a World Health Organization recommendation. It doesn't come from the DHSS, whose 1979 recommendation remains officially cancelled. This may be the first time that MAFF has ever issued an RDA for a nutrient without prior DHSS agreement. Will the DHSS have another re-think? Does the DHSS recognize the MAFF figure? By the time this book is published there may be an answer.

school children and to pregnant women were an important public health measure earlier this century. The recent withdrawal of free full-fat milk seems to have done no harm, though.

Children need more calcium than adults, and milk is a rich source of calcium. The recommendation of this report is that we should consume fewer dairy products. But in the case of milk, the solution is that skimmed and semi-skimmed milk, low in saturated fat but still rich in calcium, should be readily available for doorstep delivery.

Recommendation

• Vitamins and minerals: the recommended daily amounts for various vitamins and minerals issued by the DHSS are useful, as far as they go.

10. BABIES, YOUNG PEOPLE, THE ELDERLY

Some people in the population need special attention and can least afford to eat food that supplies calories but little or no nourishment.

Children

Could a change in the national diet to include less fats and sugars result in shorter and less healthy children?

In the last hundred years, children in Western societies have steadily grown faster and taller. This trend is associated with the increase in national wealth during the same period. For example in the USA six-year-old children were over 2½ inches taller in 1949 than they were seventy years previously, in 1880. While final adult height remained much the same during this period, in about 1950 it was being reached three or four years earlier.

However, there are indications that children's growth in Western societies has reached its maximum in the last twenty years.

Puberty

The age of puberty has steadily decreased in Western societies over the last hundred years. It looks as if the onset of puberty may be determined by reaching a certain body size; this in turn is determined mainly by the nature and quantity of food eaten. As with height, the tendency for puberty to occur at a younger and younger age seems to have slowed down in the last twenty years in Britain and elsewhere.

Is Rapid Growth Still a Good Thing?

Low birth weight, and slow growth during childhood, are both health risks. Fifty years ago and more, childhood malnutrition was a major public health problem. As a result, nutrition education emphasized the value of food that promotes growth, notably high-protein foods from animal sources, such as milk, other dairy products and meat.

This report does not recommend any reduction in protein. Rather it recommends a reduction in foods high in protein but also high in fats, and an increase in foods high in protein but low in fats. This represents a shift away from animal protein towards vegetable protein. There is no good reason to believe that such a shift would result in either shorter or less healthy children.

Rapid growth and early puberty are not necessarily beneficial. The problems with early puberty are mostly social: the earlier the age of puberty, the earlier the age of first intercourse and the greater the risk of unwanted pregnancy.

There may also be an association between early physical maturity and premature degeneration. Studies have shown that animals that grow slowly live longer. It is not known whether the same applies to people. But rapid growth is not necessarily a good thing.

The Energy Density of Food

In the Third World babies may fail to gain satisfactory weight because their diet is so bulky that their stomachs are full before they get an adequate amount of energy for growth from their food. These Third World diets may be very low in fat and very high in water content (for example, rice or maize gruels).

This problem is extremely unlikely to arise in Britain. 'Energy density' – that is, the amount of energy contained in any given volume of food – is about twice as high in Britain as in the Third World countries where this problem may arise. That is to say, British babies and children get enough energy from half the weight of food that would be adequate for a Third World child. This is because British food contains more energy in the form of fats and sugars, as well as protein.

The problem in Britain is more likely to be the reverse: children's food can be so concentrated in energy from fats and sugars and so lacking in bulk that there is room for too much energy, and the child gets fat.

Babies and Natural Food

Mother's milk is best, and breastfeeding should be encouraged. Babies should if possible be entirely breast fed for at least three months, and longer if the baby continues to grow well.

Solid food should first be given to babies some time between three and six months, depending on the child's appetite. The advantages of breast feeding should be made clear to the public. Those mothers who decide to bottlefeed should be given proper advice.

Babies should not eat solid food before the age of three

months. There is a possible link between proteins eaten in the form of solid food (milk and wheat, for instance) at a very early age and food allergies that develop in later life.

As soon as babies are ready for solids, the recommendations of this report have special application. It is most important that babies are not fed foods with added sugars or salt. A taste for sugars and salt is often established in infancy.

Cereals should not be added to bottles of milk but given to infants, mixed with milk, by spoon.

Babies and Vitamins

The recommendations here make for a bulkier diet, lower in calories, higher in nourishment. If their diet were very bulky, babies with small appetites might possibly get insufficient nourishment. There is no need for fibre supplements for children.

Adequate vitamin intake is essential for babies and young children. In particular, low birth-weight babies, Asian children, children whose vitamin D level is thought to be low (children whose sunlight exposure is infrequent), and any baby who is brought up on doorstep milk*, should be given children's vitamin drops, available from health visitors or the doctor, or a suitable over-the-counter alternative. Children must not be given more than one 'dose' of vitamin D (because large amounts can be toxic).

Adolescents and Deranged Eating Habits

Obsessive starvation known as anorexia nervosa, and 'bingeing' followed by vomiting, known as bulimia, are common disorders among adolescent girls. One estimate is that one in 100 girls over the age of sixteen is anorexic.

---

*The DHSS advises that no baby under the age of 6 months be given doorstep cow's milk, which is unsuitable for the human infant. Health visitors can advise about the best alternatives to breast feeding.

Girls who starve themselves are liable to be deficient in various nutrients. The problem will grow worse if they become pregnant. Also, many girls believe that starchy foods, being carbohydrate-rich, must be avoided. But at the same time they may snack obsessively on foods heavy in fats and sugars. It is particularly important that in periods of growth, such as adolescence, people eat nutritious food. The recommendations of this report are therefore especially relevant to 'slimming' girls.

Other adolescents, both boys and girls, may eat adequate food at school and at home, and also eat and drink large amounts of snacks. More and more, nowadays, adolescents eat snacks rather than meals. It is therefore important that snacks that are low in fats, sugars and salt are manufactured.

The Elderly and Exercise

As people get older they tend to lose lean tissue, including muscle, and gain fat. Because lean tissue is lost, the speed at which their bodies burn energy (the metabolic rate) slows down. As a result ageing people are liable to gain fat while eating less. They may therefore develop nutritional deficiencies.

Everybody should stay active throughout life. This is the best way to preserve lean tissue and a good appetite without gaining fat.

The elderly also have special need of nourishing food.

Ethnic Minorities and Vitamin D

Gross deficiency of vitamin D is the cause of rickets. Deficiency of vitamin D is also a cause of osteomalacia (weakening of the bones). Rickets is known to occur in schoolchildren of Asian origin in Britain. Osteomalacia is common in elderly women, including those of Asian origin.

The recommendation is that Asian schoolchildren should be

given vitamin D supplements. This is best done within their community.

Recommendation

• Special groups: the recommendations in the report apply to everybody. The special care of babies, children, adolescents, pregnant women, ethnic minorities and the elderly make it all the more important that they eat nourishing food.

11. THE GOALS: HOW TO PUT THE BRITISH DIET RIGHT

The long-term goals for the 1980s and 1990s are as follows:

• The recommendations are for the population as a whole, not for 'at risk groups'. We are all at risk from the typical British diet.

• The recommendations are for average intakes for the population, and not for each individual person.

• Usually, overweight people should not eat less, but exercise more. At the same time they should change their eating patterns.

• Smoking is more dangerous than overweight. At the same time, ex-smokers should also exercise more and change their eating patterns.

• Fats: consumption should be cut by one quarter, to 30 per cent of total energy intake from the present level of about 38 per cent.

• Saturated fats: consumption should be cut by nearly one half, to 10 per cent of total energy intake from the present level of 18 per cent.

- Polyunsaturated fats: there is no recommendation to increase the amount eaten. The proportion of polyunsaturates to saturates eaten will rise because of the cut in saturated fats.

- Cholesterol: there is no recommendation to cut the amount eaten.

- Sugars: consumption should be cut by one half, to 10 per cent of total energy intake from the present level of 20 per cent.

- Sugars in snacks: consumption should be no more than half total sugar intake, or 4 to 5 per cent of total energy intake.

- Fibre: consumption should be increased by one half, to 30 grams a day from the present level of 20 grams a day. This should take the form of whole food: cereals, and also vegetables and fruit.

- Salt: consumption should be cut by about one half, to 5 grams a day from the present level of 8–12 grams.

- Alcohol: consumption should be cut by one third, to 4 per cent of total energy intake from the present level of 6 per cent.

- Protein: there is no recommendation to change the amount eaten. The amount of animal protein should fall; the amount of vegetable protein should rise.

- Vitamins and minerals: the recommended daily amounts for various vitamins and minerals issued by the DHSS are useful, as far as they go.

- Special groups: the recommendations apply to everybody. Special care of babies, children, adolescents, pregnant women, ethnic minorities and the elderly is within the context of these recommendations.

- Food labelling: there is a need for clear and informative food labelling with details of calories, energy, fats, saturated fats, sugars and salt content of foods.

The Goals Summarized

A summary of the recommended goals follows. Those for protein, fats, sugars, starches and alcohol are expressed as percentages of total calorie intake. (The figure for starches is derived from the other figures; the figures for sugars and starches are rounded up and down.) The figures for fibre (contained in cereal, vegetables and fruit) and for salt are expressed as grams per day. Current figures are also given for comparison:

	Change	Current	Recommended
		per cent of energy	
Protein	No change	11	11
Fats	Down by one quarter	38	30
Sugars	Down by one half	20	10
Starches	Up by more than one half	25	45
Alcohol	Down by one third	6	4
Total		100	100
		grams per day	
Fibre	Up by one half	20	30
Salt	Down by about one half	8–12	5

Healthy Food is Also Delicious

The national diet recommended here contains less fats, sugars, and salt. It is and should be delicious. The proportions of protein, fats, sugars and starches recommended here are traditional in many cultures whose food is well known to be delicious: Mediterranean countries, for example. In other countries the diet is varied and attractive while containing perhaps one third of the fats we consume.

When the recommended diet is expressed in terms of menus and recipes (as it already is by community dieticians and in many popular magazines) it should prove more, rather than less, varied and attractive than the food we eat now.

The Interim Goals

These changes in the national diet cannot be made immediately. They require changes in government and EEC regulations, the support of government and industry, and a shift in the public attitude to food and health. Most expert groups that have worked on dietary change estimate that fifteen years will be needed to achieve the long-term goals.

The recommended short-term goals for the 1980s consist of about one third of the recommended long-term changes. This seems reasonable and modest, and well within today's broad scientific consensus. The short-term programme is as follows.

- Fats: consumption to be cut by 10 per cent. Saturated fats: consumption to be cut by 15 per cent. Polyunsaturated fats: consumption to be increased by one quarter, to 5 per cent of energy intake (from the present low level of 4 per cent: a small increase in terms of volume).

Interim measures involve small cuts in consumption of saturated fats in meat, dairy products, biscuits and cakes; and an increase in consumption of some margarines and vegetable oils.

- Sugars: consumption to be cut by 10 per cent. Sugars in snacks: consumption to be cut sharply to the recommended long-term levels.

- Calories. Usually people should not eat less, but exercise more.

The shift from foods high in fats and sugars to whole foods

involves increasing the consumption of bread, potatoes, vegetables and fruit by about one quarter, or a little more. The main single increase should be to eat more bread, notably wholemeal and brown bread. We should eat perhaps half as much bread again (an extra 70 to 100 calories a day).

- Fibre: consumption to be increased by 25 per cent.

- Salt: consumption to be cut by 10 per cent.

- Alcohol: consumption to be cut by 10 per cent.

The logic of these interim changes is that they can be made by individuals, and are not designed to make significant demands on food manufacturers. It will take time, for example, for manufacturers to decrease the volume of sugar and salt in their products. A summary of the interim goals follows.

	Change	*Current*	*For the 1980s*
		per cent of energy	
Protein	No change	11	11
Fats	Down by one tenth	38	34
Sugars	Down by one tenth	20	18
Starches	Up by one quarter	25	32
Alcohol	Down by one sixth	6	5
Total		100	100
		grams per day	
Fibre	Up by one quarter	20	25
Salt	Down by one tenth	8–12	7–11

Watching the Changes Work

Samples of the population should be studied regularly to ascertain changes in health and in the risk of disease as the dietary changes are put into practice. (This could be done as part of the National Food Survey carried out by the Ministry of Agriculture, Fisheries and Food).

Measurements to be taken from such samples should include weight, blood pressure and blood profile.

12. WHAT GOVERNMENT & INDUSTRY CAN DO

National eating habits can only change substantially with support from institutions, industry and government.

Meals served in schools, canteens, hospitals and other institutions should have a lower content of fats, sugars and salt. And cookery instruction, for example in schools and colleges, should emphasize not only that meals low in fats, sugars and salt are healthy but also that, well prepared, they look attractive and taste delicious.

The food and agriculture industries, together with government, have a special responsibility. Some necessary developments are:

- Breeding lean animals
- Changes in government standards designed to encourage farmers to breed lean animals
- Reduction in the fat content of processed meat products, such as sausages and pies
- Better labelling of food: labels should include details of calories, fats, saturated fats, sugars and salt content of all foods
- Avoidance of any legislation that has the effect of encouraging consumption of fats, sugars, salt or alcohol
- Strengthening of the laws governing the composition of food

Looking to the Future

If the food industry and the farmers recognize that doctors and scientists are for practical purposes sure that changes in the national diet are necessary to improve health and prevent disease, then they can plan to help bring about the goals set out here.

Much can be done by manufacturing and promoting food that is healthy (low in fats, sugars and salt), reasonably priced and widely available.

Much more can be done by those professionally concerned with food and health working in partnership with food suppliers, and manufacturers and retailers.

13. HOW THE REPORT WAS WRITTEN

The NACNE report is a synthesis of the recommendations of various expert committees set up by the DHSS and the Royal College of Physicians in recent years, together with a recent World Health Organization report.

It is recognized that some individual scientists may hold different views from those on which this report is based.

In preparing the report, a very large number of interested parties, expert groups and individuals, and scientific and medical papers, have been consulted. The report is a collaborative national effort that seeks to identify what is wrong with the diet of the British people as a whole, including the typical average diet, and to state goals for change.

Goals are given for the next fifteen years, for the 1980s and 1990s; and interim goals, for the 1980s, are also given.

These targets are scientifically based, feasible and worthwhile. They provide everybody professionally concerned with food and health education with realistic guidelines.

Much now needs to be done. Partners in the necessary changes include government, the Department of Health and Social Security (DHSS), the Ministry of Agriculture, Fisheries and Food (MAFF), the Health Education Council, the food industry and the farmers.

The National Advisory Committee on Nutrition Education looks forward to the national debate that its report should stimulate.

The Status of the Report

The NACNE report on *Proposals for Nutritional Guidelines for Health Education in Britain*, published by the Health Education Council in September 1983, is intended for use by organizations concerned directly or indirectly with health and nutrition education, and not for the general public.

The Food Scandal is intended for the general public, as well as for dieticians, doctors, health visitors, school teachers, manufacturers, distributors and retailers of food, caterers and others professionally concerned with the quality of food.

The NACNE report does not represent the individual views of Professor James; nor of the panel of experts who, with Professor James, did the initial work on the report; nor of the large number of organizations and individuals consulted as the report was compiled. The report presents a consensus of views primarily derived from government reports and from other major expert committees.

Sources Used for the NACNE Report

The eight main sources for the NACNE report are:

a. *Eating for Health,* Department of Health and Social Security— DHSS, 1978, 1979: HMSO
b. *Diet and Coronary Heart Disease,* DHSS Report on Health and Social Subjects No. 7, 1974: HMSO
c. *Prevention of Coronary Artery Disease,* Joint Report of the Royal College of Physicians and the British Cardiac Society, 1976
d. *Medical Aspects of Dietary Fibre,* Report of the Royal College of Physicians, 1981: Pitman
e. *Recommended Daily Amounts of Food Energy and Nutrients for Groups of People in the United Kingdom,* DHSS Report on Health and Social Subjects No. 15, 1981: HMSO
f. *Avoiding Heart Attacks,* DHSS Report, 1981: HMSO
g. *Prevention of Coronary Heart Disease,* World Health Organization, 1982: WHO
h. *Obesity,* Report of the Royal College of Physicians, 1983: RCP

PART 2

Questions and Answers about Food and Health

Since the NACNE report became public knowledge in 1983, the authors of this book have been asked many questions about its contents and meaning – by colleagues and friends, doctors and dieticians, politicians and teachers; by members of the public who have written many letters to us, concerned for their health and for the health of their families; and when interviewed for television, radio, newspapers and magazines. Since first publication of *The Food Scandal* the book itself has generated interest. Here are thirty of the questions asked or reactions received, with the answers.

1. Can the Basic Message about Food and Health be Expressed in One Sentence?

Yes. First, it is a question of realizing what everybody all over the world and throughout history has understood, perhaps with the exception only of people in the West in recent years: the quality of health, and therefore the quality of life, depends upon the quality of food. Ironically, this fundamental truth should be most obvious to us now in the West, since we are shielded from the mass epidemics of infections that ravage crowded towns without adequate sanitation.

The one sentence message is as follows. For good health, eat whole, fresh food; and prefer food of vegetable origin.

2. What Do the Scientists Say About Food and Health?

The message of the NACNE report in 1983, of the McGovern report issued in the USA in 1977, and of statements issued by expert committees in Western countries, given the brief to make recommendations designed to improve the health of the people in these countries, is as follows. To prevent disease, eat less fats, sugars and salt; and eat more fibre.

3. That Doesn't Sound Much Like Fun. Is there Another Way of Expressing this Message?

Representatives of the vested interests that oppose plans for a more healthy national diet, have had some success when they say that the recommendations of NACNE and of other expert committees are dull, negative and unpalatable. The boffins (it is suggested) are telling us to stop eating the food we enjoy and, instead, to munch bran or stalks.

The NACNE report was written to be read by public health professionals, who are mostly concerned with the prevention of disease as distinct from the promotion of positive health (even though these two aims are really as indivisible as the two sides of the same coin). Also, the NACNE recommendations rely mainly on recommendations of other expert committees, which in turn rely on many hundreds of scientific studies that establish, beyond reasonable doubt, that fats, sugars and salt (eaten in the great quantities they are eaten in the West) cause diseases; and that fibre (eaten in greater quantities than now eaten in the West) protects against diseases. It is vitally important that health professionals (especially doctors, who are not taught nutrition) should appreciate the fundamental importance of food to health; hence the need for the careful accumulation of detailed scientific evidence supporting the NACNE recommendations. To a lay person this process, and the language of medical research, does seem negative, and often dull, too.

It is also true that eating fibre by itself (in the form of bran) is a glum business. People do not sprinkle bran on their food for fun. No poet has attempted an ode to fibre. Bulky stools are not the stuff that dreams are made on.

Hence the positive message of this book, which is indeed a translation of the message of the NACNE report into everyday language: for good health, eat whole, fresh food; and prefer food of vegetable origin.

4. It's All About Avoiding Heart Attacks and Obesity, Isn't It?

No, it isn't.

It is true that diseases of the blood vessels are the direct cause of more deaths in Britain (and other Western countries) than any other group of diseases. These 'cardiovascular' diseases cause around 250,000 deaths in Britain every year, from heart attacks, strokes, and other fatal conditions elsewhere in the body. Cardiovascular diseases are also the major single cause of premature death (under the age of 65). They usually cause at least some degree of disability and suffering before death.

Consequently, cardiovascular diseases are of special interest to doctors, and massive resources have been spent in attempts to identify their causes. For example, a recent project in the USA which established beyond reasonable doubt that raised blood cholesterol increases the risk of heart attacks, cost $165 million.

So, given the scale of the public health problem represented by heart disease and other cardiovascular diseases, and given that they are diet-related diseases largely preventable by eating healthy food, it is understandable that they are given prominence in expert committee reports. Four of the eight reports on which the NACNE report itself mainly relies are concerned with the prevention specifically of heart disease, and another, *Diet and Cardiovascular Disease*, was published by the DHSS in July 1984.

It is also true that overweight and obesity are, together, often identified as the biggest public health problem in Britain (and other Western countries). Over one third of all British adults are overweight. Fat people, women especially, suffer professionally, socially and sexually, and are taught that being fat is their fault. Generally speaking, fat people are unfit even by the low 'normal' standard of a society in which most people are sedentary; and when people continue to gain weight and eventually become even obese the quality of their lives, generally, declines. It is no fun being fat.

From the medical point of view, overweight increases the risk of suffering from many common diseases, including various cancers, arthritis, gall-bladder disease, varicose veins and high blood pressure; and overweight, diabetes and heart disease are closely related to one another.

Most people assume that overweight is caused by eating too much food – or, frankly, by greed – and that the way to prevent and cure overweight is to eat less food. For this reason doctors are often exasperated by patients who ask to be treated for overweight. Likewise, popular dieting books, superficially different from one another, are in fact mostly based on the 'calorie-cutting' principle, as are most slimming organizations and 'health farms'.

But it is now understood that while greed (or compulsive eating) is of course liable to cause gain of fat, generally speaking fat people do not eat proportionately more than slim people. The main causes of overweight are lack of exercise and eating the wrong kind of food, and the way to prevent and cure overweight is to eat the right kind of food and also to take regular vigorous exercise.

This vital re-think about the cause of overweight is reason enough for it to be given prominence in expert committee reports. One of the eight reports on which the NACNE report itself mainly relies is *Obesity*, published by the Royal College of Physicians in 1983. This is the best source of modern medical thinking about overweight. The two leading British authorities on obesity, Professor James himself, and Dr John Garrow (now chairman of JACNE, the successor to NACNE) were prominent members of the Royal College committee that produced this report.

So there is good reason for any expert report on food and health to pay a lot of attention to the prevention of heart attacks and also of obesity.

That said, the NACNE report also shows that the food we eat in the West is a prime underlying cause of many other diseases and disorders. These range from the disagreeable (tooth decay and constipation, as well as overweight), to the disabling (diabetes, gall-bladder disease, brittle bones) to the deadly (various cancers, as well as heart attacks and strokes).

It is also quite wrong to suppose that Western food is liable to damage our health only in middle and old age. Apart from tooth decay, constipation and overweight, the food we eat is a prime cause of diseases and disorders of infants, children, adolescents, pregnant women and young adults. Bad food can damage mental as well as physical health. Employed people who eat well are less likely to suffer from the 'thank God it's Friday' syndrome.

Everybody will gain from learning about food and health.

5. So I Can't Eat Anything, Then . . .

The English have a habit of making their jokes seriously, and a standard quip, half flippant, half anxious, made when the authors of this book are asked about food, is something along the lines of 'I suppose you think that everything's bad for me' or 'If I was to believe what you say I'd have to starve'.

If every diet-related disease had a completely different cause, there would be reason for people either to become neurotic about what they ate, or else adopt a 'to hell with it!' attitude, and pay no attention to what they ate. Shops cause some confusion, by stocking slimming foods on one counter, diabetic foods on another, 'health' foods on another, and all the other foods (for people with no problems?) on the other shelves. Newspapers make things worse, by publishing stories suggesting that one food is a killer, another a cure-all, without proper explanation or rationale (like doctors, medical correspondents are not taught nutrition). Slimmers are trained to fear food by the competing and contradictory claims of the regimes published in magazines and books. And, meanwhile, the manufacturers of highly processed foods spend big money advertising their products. In 1983 one firm, Mars Ltd, spent £34 million on advertising in Britain.

But not every diet, and not every food, is a significant cause of disease. The good news carried by the NACNE report, which is also a warning, is that all the evidence points to the same elements of our diet being the problem. Western diseases are caused by Western food; that is to say, by those constituents of our diet that makes it different from non-Western diets: fats, sugars, and salt, in the quantity these are now eaten on average in Britain, together with alcohol.

6. Our Ancestors Seemed to Manage Perfectly Well Without all this Preoccupation with Food

Many of our ancestors had other problems: famine, pestilence and war, for instance. More recently, until well into this century, millions of poor people and children suffered from deficiency diseases caused by wretched, monotonous diets and in particular by eating no fruit and only (often half-rotten) root vegetables in the winter months. The causes of deficiency diseases were not well understood until after vitamins were identified as vital to health, notably in the period 1910–1930. Captain Scott probably died from scurvy, readily avoidable if he had carried or stored sufficient citrus fruit and potatoes.

Many of our ancestors did not manage perfectly well. This book is not a celebration of medieval or Victorian days. Frozen food and the refrigerator are great benefits. Almost every supermarket contains plenty of good food, if you know how to choose and pick. Street markets, greengrocers and fishmongers have not died out yet. Cheap travel has shown us exotic cuisines; the twilight of Empire has brought exotic food even to the back streets (beware, though, the greasy travesties that we have taught the Indians, Chinese and Cypriots to serve to us).

We have a lot of food to be thankful for, and most readers of this book can eat better than maybe at any other time of British history.

The issue is choice. Our ancestors did not have much of a choice, most of the time, and when they did, usually were not aware of the long-term consequences of their choices. The knowledge that the food we eat in the West is the main single underlying cause of most of the diseases we suffer and die from, is new. It gives us freedom because it gives us the choice to improve, maybe even transform our health; to put more life in our years even if not more years in our life. It gives us more responsibility, not only for ourselves, but also for our children.

Sometimes people prefer to evade choice; it can be painful. A mother whose child's teeth are rotten will not enjoy learning that the disease was caused by sweet drinks given to the child in infancy. An executive does not want to hear that two of his friends had heart attacks in early middle age because of the lunches and dinners he still enjoys. A husband whose wife is crippled after a stroke will find the idea hard to take that one cause of her grievous condition may well have been salty food. Almost all senior politicians, and almost all senior doctors, are middle-aged men: bluntly, most of them do not want to know about food and health. It's worth remembering, too, that almost all directors in the food industry, and big landowners, are middle-aged men. These have three compelling reasons to reject the evidence that connects food, health and disease. First, as with politicians and doctors, fifty or sixty years is a long time to have been digging your grave with your teeth, and a hard time to face the fact that, unknowing, you have made the wrong food choices. Second, people in food and farming do not want to believe that their business harms people – who would? Third, and this alas may be the most compelling reason of all, unhealthy food makes the most money. Much talk against the messages of the NACNE report is money talking. Most changes towards a healthy national diet, of the type our ancestors tended to eat when they had the chance, will be made by people who do not have an investment in insisting that the current British diet is healthy. People concerned for their children may lead the way.

7. What's So Special About the NACNE Report?

Scientists, doctors and nutritionists among them, are trained to specialize, and to make statements only about 'their subject'. This system of knowing more and more about less and less is dangerous; knowledge can drive out wisdom.

Doctors still enjoy extraordinary prestige. Children who dream of becoming doctors read of Livingstone and Schweitzer, Pasteur and Fleming. And it may be true that most advances in science and medicine are made by idealists and campaigners. However, most of the power, money and glory in medicine is gained by people morally and spiritually no different from the rest of us (is it reasonable to expect otherwise?) Data accumulation and classification, together with ingenious and sophisticated repair jobs, are what gain the research grants, publicity, big budgets and professorships. An old crocks run of every British heart transplant patient from Westminster Bridge, if not to Brighton then perhaps to the Elephant and Castle, would get front page treatment from most national newspapers.

In this environment any well-founded expert report on the prevention of disease is remarkable. In so far as medicine is a business, prevention is bad for business.

In the summer of 1984, much publicity was given to the expert report *Diet and Cardiovascular Disease* produced for the DHSS by the COMA panel on medical aspects of food policy. From the medical point of view there was very little new in the report; it was almost entirely a repetition, and a cautious repetition, of four previous reports published since 1974 on the prevention of heart disease on which the NACNE report had relied. From the political point of view *Diet and Cardiovascular Disease* was and is important, because the official government line, while disowning the NACNE report, in 1983 and 1984, was repeatedly to state that the COMA report was the one on which government policy would be based.

The COMA panel duly reported that dietary fats are a major cause of cardiovascular diseases and that, in order to prevent these diseases, the British people should eat less fats and, notably, less saturated and processed fats. Moreover, the food industry should, in the view of the panel, label processed foods with their percentage of fats, saturated fats and polyunsaturated fats content.

So the good thing about the *Diet and Cardiovascular Disease* report is that at last the British government has acknowledged the modern medical consensus view that major Western diseases are diet-related; that the average British diet is a major cause of heart disease; and that the food industry should make changes designed to encourage a healthier national diet.

But the conventional thing about the report is that it deals with only one group of Western diseases (albeit pandemic in Britain) and, characteristically, settles on one dietary cause almost to the exclusion of any other. The subject? Heart disease. The victim? Middle-aged Western man. The villain? Saturated fats. Life and death is reduced to a version of Cluedo.

The great thing about the NACNE report is that it has vision. It is not specialized. It is not an advance on the McGovern report, and it is less remarkable a piece of thinking than classic text books on food and health written in the last thirty years by Surgeon-Captain T. L. Cleave, Dr Hugh Trowell, and Dr Denis Burkitt. But it is the first general statement on food and health recently published in Britain that demonstrates that the issue is not one item of our diet, nor one disease (however common), but Western food and Western disease in general. It paints a picture that we can all recognize.

8. Which Diseases Are Diet-related?

The NACNE report mentions a large number of diseases and disorders. Of these it identifies a dozen as being certainly or almost certainly not only diet-related, but also caused by too much fat, sugar and/or salt, or not enough fibre. Most of these are diseases that usually show themselves in middle age.

Diet-related diseases are known either as diseases of over-consumption, or as diseases of under-nutrition. The most obvious example of a disease of over-consumption is obesity, when (untypically) it is caused by greed. The most obvious example of a disease of under-nutrition is emaciation caused by starvation – eating far too little of everything.

Diseases can, however, be caused by over-consumption of one specific part of the diet: and 'over-consumption' can mean the amount that we in Britain consider to be normal. It can even mean less than the national average amount eaten. For example, tooth decay is caused by eating too much processed sugar, and would not be eliminated in Britain if the national average consumption of sugar was cut in half.

There again, diseases can be caused by under-nutrition of one specific part of the diet. For example, constipation is caused by not eating enough fibre. Other diseases come from a combination of over-consumption and under-nutrition. A diet high in fats and sugars is almost bound to be a diet low in fibre, vitamins and minerals.

The diseases and disorders identified in the NACNE report as being caused by over-consumption of fats, sugars and/or salt, and/or by under-nutrition of fibre, are as follows:

Over-consumption		Under-nutrition
fats	cancer of large bowel (colon)	fibre
	constipation	fibre
fats, sugars	diabetes*	
	diverticular disease	fibre
fats, sugars	gall-bladder disease*	fibre
fats	heart disease*	
fats, salt	high blood pressure*	
	irritable bowel	fibre
fats, sugars	overweight, obesity	fibre
fats, salt	strokes	
sugars	tooth decay	

*also associated with overweight and obesity.

There is a pattern to be seen in this list. Of the disabling and deadly diseases, over-consumption of fats tends to cause diseases of the cardiovascular system (of the heart and blood vessels) and under-nutrition of fibre tends to cause diseases of the alimentary tract (the gut; specifically, the lower gut).

The NACNE report also identifies other diseases of over-consumption or under-nutrition with other diet-related causes. For example, in excess, alcohol poisons the body in general and causes liver disease in particular. The higher the level of consumption the greater the risk to the individual. As well as rickets and scurvy (not unknown in Britain, but now uncommon) osteomalacia and osteoporosis (weakening of the bones, very common in old women) are identified as caused in part by under-nutrition of a vitamin. And reference is made to the well-documented view that neural tube defects in babies (the best known of which is spina bifida) are also caused in part by vitamin under-nutrition. So the list of diet-related diseases increases:

Over-consumption		*Under-nutrition*
alcohol	cirrhosis of liver	
	neural tube defects	vitamin (folic acid)
	osteomalacia*	vitamin D
	osteoporosis*	vitamin D

*also caused by lack of exercise.

9. Is That the Lot?

No, it isn't. It is certain that the NACNE report has omitted many diet-related diseases. It lists diseases as diet-related only when they have been identified as such by expert medical and scientific committees in Britain, working either to the DHSS or else to the Royal College of Physicians. (Use is also made of one World Health Organization document.) A report which is essentially a synthesis of other reports is necessarily cautious; and Professor James has said that he was, therefore, astonished that successive drafts of the NACNE report were blocked by the DHSS for over two years.

In March 1984, the US Department of Health, Education and Welfare (the American equivalent of the DHSS) stated as national policy that many cancers are diet-related and that the best approach to these cancers is prevention. This followed major statements made by the US National Academy of Sciences (a body somewhat like the Royal Society or the Royal College of Physicians). The eminent researcher Sir Richard Doll, emeritus professor of medicine at Oxford University, who jointly established the connection between cigarette smoking and lung cancer, has stated that Western food is the main single underlying cause of cancers; a bigger killer than smoking, and a much bigger killer than chemical pollution. If NACNE was reporting now, or had reported in 1984, it would have taken account of the new and formidable evidence linking Western food and various cancers.

Some common conditions, known to be associated with diet-related diseases identified in the NACNE report, are nevertheless not named in the report. These include angina (an aspect of heart disease) and piles and varicose veins (complications of constipation).

Ulcers of the alimentary tract are also known to be diet-related diseases, but they are not popular subjects for research, because nobody has yet been able to identify a specific dietary cause; like many other diseases their underlying cause may well be Western food in general, not any particular element of the diet. Some diet-related diseases are not specifically Western diseases, either. The Japanese eat more salt than we do, and suffer and die not only more from high blood pressure and strokes than we do, but also, in some parts of Japan, from more stomach cancer. Cancer of the gullet (oesophagus), too, has been linked with food intake in several countries.

So the list of diet-related diseases, for which there is strong scientific evidence, increases further:

Over-consumption		*Under-nutrition*
fats	angina	
fats, sugars?	cancer of breast	
fats?	cancer of pancreas	
salt	cancer of stomach	
	piles	fibre
sugars?	kidney stones	
fats?, sugars?	ulcer of intestine	fibre?
fats?, sugars?	ulcer of stomach	fibre?
	varicose veins	fibre

10. Is *That* the Lot?

No. There are a great number more diseases that are caused by the food we eat. The evidence for the causal connection is not yet accepted as firm, for various reasons. 'Firm' evidence, to scientists, means evidence that has been reproduced again and again: a recent study of the links between processed sugars in food and kidney stone formation remains the speciality of one man (Professor Norman Blacklock of Manchester University Medical School). Some other elements of the food we eat are well known internationally to be vital, but have not yet been properly accepted as such in Britain; so despite the fact that two British researchers, Dr Hugh Sinclair, followed by Professor Michael Crawford, are world authorities on essential fats, discussion of essential fats and their role in protection against disease is still more or less confined to expert medical journals. Likewise, hypoglycaemia (abnormal swings in blood sugar causing abnormal swings in mental and physical function) and hyperactivity (bizarre behaviour, notably found in children) are not yet accepted as genuine disorders in Britain, despite being well accepted as major problems in other Western countries.

The NACNE report says nothing about food additives or food allergy, and makes no reference to the real possibility that various conditions of childhood (acne, eczema, migraine, and psoriaris, as well as hyperactivity) are diet-related, as well as other conditions (asthma and hay fever, for example) that can persist into adult life. And there is almost no mention of 'female' conditions that are probably diet-related (anorexia nervosa, bulimia, breast pain, pre-menstrual tension).

The following diseases probably have the typical British diet as an underlying cause:

Over-consumption		*Under-nutrition*
	appendicitis	fibre
	arthritis	essential fats?
additives	eczema*	
alcohol	foetal alcohol syndrome	
sugars	gout	

Over-consumption		Under-nutrition
	hiatus hernia	fibre?
addititives	hyperactivity*	
sugars	hypoglycaemia**	
additives	migraine and allergies*	
	multiple sclerosis?	essential fats?
	rheumatoid arthritis?	essential fats?

*can also be caused by cereals, cow's milk and other foods.
**can also be caused by other foods.

A question mark placed against a disease or a dietary cause means that there is good reason to suspect the disease is diet-related, or suspect a dietary cause, but that the area remains speculative.

Is that the lot *now*, then? No, it isn't. The diseases listed above are those now known (or in a few cases suspected) to be diet-related in the sense that they have the typical British diet as a, or the, major single underlying cause. This does not of course mean that they are wholly caused by the food we eat. Heart disease and all its complications is also caused by smoking and lack of exercise, for instance (and a number of relatively rare types of heart disease are not to do with diet).

As research is extended into new areas the list of diet-related diseases will grow. But it is reasonable to say that all non-infectious diseases have unhealthy food as a contributory cause, even though the food may only be one cause among others.

It is also reasonable to say that since unhealthy food weakens the immune system, it reduces the resistance to infections. Two people may be exposed to the same bug: the person who is better nourished is liable to recover quicker, suffer a milder infection, or not show any sign of infection.

The same point also applies to trauma of any kind. After a wound caused by a burn, say, or a car accident, or surgery, the body in effect operates an emergency service, rushing its own stores of nourishment to the site of injury. The person whose body tissues are highly saturated with vitamins and minerals from healthy food, will recover faster, and in a severe crisis is more likely to survive. In such emergencies knowledgeable doctors inject highly concentrated cocktails of nutrients into the bloodstream ('parenteral nutrition') to supplement the stores already in the body. Less is known about mental trauma, caused by death of a spouse, say, or long-term unemployment, but it is certain that good food is crucial to mental as well as physical health.

11. So What Does That Leave? Only Murders and Car Crashes?

No. Most murders and many deaths on the road occur under the influence of alcohol.

12. When You've Got to Go, You've Got to Go. Isn't a Heart Attack a Clean end?

When we think of our own deaths, we would all like to die in peace and without pain, full of years and experience.

Death from a heart attack can indeed strike suddenly, without warning, 'out of the blue'.

Two out of five of all men in Britain who die before the age of 65, die of a heart attack. Even when these deaths are sudden, they are premature and likely to be a savage blow to the families of the dead man. This type of unexpected death, whether in bed, in the street, or on the lavatory, is also liable to lack dignity: unintentionally, it can be in effect a selfish end, at any age.

But most deaths from heart disease come after years – twenty-five years, maybe – of slowing down, discomfort, pain, associated diseases such as obesity and diabetes, hospital, and operations. The actual end may be quick – though many people survive several heart attacks. But the process of the development of heart disease is slow and usually depressing and disabling many years before death.

The same is true of strokes. Anybody who has lived with a loved one who has survived a serious stroke, with the loss of much mental and physical function, knows that strokes are not a happy approach to death. The death-in-life suffered by a stroke victim with irreversible brain damage is cruel beyond words.

Cancers are not, of course, seen by anybody as a favourite cause of death. Britain may turn out to be the last Western country officially to accept that most common cancers are diet-related diseases.

13. Would You Rather Die of a Heart Attack Aged 70 or of Senile Dementia Aged 80?

Watch for this question. It often comes up in media debates about food and health. It is a question that has been worked out by people who are paid by the saturated fats and sugars industries to represent their interests in public.

It's rather a last-ditch defence of saturated fats and sugars and salt. Effectively, it's saying: 'OK, let's agree that saturated fats, sugars and salt are killers. But they're clean killers. Indeed they're mercy killers. The choice is living the average lifespan and keeling over in good health; or dragging out an extra ten years of incompetence and incontinence, out of your mind, a burden to yourself and your family.'

This argument is rubbish. Chairmen and managing directors of the fats and sugars industries are not noted for snuffing themselves out at three score years and ten. Deaths from heart attacks (or strokes or cancers) are usually not clean deaths at any age. And there is no evidence that dementia ('senile' or otherwise) is an inevitable consequence of old age. Of course it is true that we slow down with age; generally, the process starts around the age of twenty-five and accelerates around forty-five and more so at about sixty-five. But this slowing down is not dementia. The miserable old people, bed-ridden or sitting in chairs all day, at home or in 'a home' are not suffering from old age; they are suffering from despair, neglect, and almost certainly, vile food.

One type of dementia, known sometimes as 'premature senile dementia' and medically as Alzheimer's disease, which is quite common in Britain, and tends to become obvious in late middle age, is now suspected to be caused in part by chronic poisoning from the toxic mineral, aluminium. Poisoning from toxic minerals is accelerated by an unhealthy diet.

14. All This Sounds Very Gloomy and Doomy. What's the Good News?

The good news is that healthy food is the best way to positive good health; to the sense of well-being that we so often assume is lost with childhood.

Eat well and you are more likely – in time, much more likely – to wake up and look forward to enjoying the day; to enjoy yourself; and to have the energy to be a pleasure for the people in your life.

15. If All This is True, Why Haven't I heard it Before?

Doctors are not taught nutrition. The subject is not on the syllabus for medical students (who learn scraps of information about nutrition as only of passing interest). No medical school in Britain yet has a nutrition department. In the late 1930s the British medical establishment believed that the relevant discoveries about human nutrition and health had all, by then, been made, so thereafter nutrition became a backwater. Nutritionists are commonly confused with dieticians, who are commonly thought to be a sort of auxiliary nurse. Most people trained as nutritionists work in food science and technology, or in the food industry. The subject of nutrition has carried little prestige in the past forty years.

Since the Second World War doctors in the USA have become increasingly interested in the causal connections between Western food and Western diseases. The pioneers were heart disease specialists like Professor Jeremiah Stamler, and epidemiologists like Professor Ancel Keys (both still active) who succeeded in persuading the younger generations of doctors of the link between saturated fats and heart disease. In the 1970s similar work started on the causal connection between Western food and cancers. The culmination of this work was the publication in 1977 of the McGovern report, *Dietary Goals for the United States*, which continues to receive massive attention from the media in the USA and probably more than any other single influence has convinced the American nation of the vital links between food and health. A poll taken in 1981 showed that two thirds of all people in the USA had by then changed their eating habits for health reasons.

No such general change has taken place in Britain, either within the medical profession or publicly. It is now well known that the UK has the highest rates of deaths from heart disease in the world, and that these rates are not significantly dropping. It is less well known that the UK also has very high rates of birth defects, tooth decay, multiple sclerosis and cancers, to name just four causes of largely preventable suffering. Moreover, the incidence of diseases such as these tends to be highest in Scotland, Northern Ireland and Wales, where the greatest amount of highly processed food is eaten.

Why is change happening in the USA – and in Canada, Australia, and most of the European countries with higher rates of Western diseases – but not in the UK?

The cynical answer to the question 'Why haven't I heard all this before?' is 'In whose interests is it to tell you?' Currently the food industry makes more profit from highly processed food than from whole, fresh food. The drug industry depends on ill people; the slimming industry depends on fat people. However many people there are who work in these titanic industries who are genuinely concerned for the health of their fellow men, women and children, economic forces are against them.

What about government? The Department of Health is also the Department of Social Security; and civil servants who work for the SS division of the DHSS point out that longer-lived people will cost the Exchequer more money in old-age pensions. The Ministry of Food is also the Ministry of Agriculture and Fisheries; and civil servants who work for MAFF point out that a national healthy food policy would be against the current interests of the food industry and food manufacturers. The European Common Agricultural Policy subsidizes the production of fat meat and fat milk and dairy produce – and the result is the European butter mountain and milk lake.

The media – television, radio, newspapers, magazines – do not have the vested interest in highly processed food that food manufacturers themselves have. But the food industry is a massive advertiser: the sugar and chocolate confectionery firms alone spent £400 million on advertising in 1983 – forty times the total annual budget of the Health Education Council. Food manufacturers also pay for most of the messages sent out to the media, and to doctors, health professionals and schools. The British Nutrition Foundation may sound like the Ford Foundation, but it is in fact wholly funded by the food industry, and seeks to advise the public about food through the media. And anybody who imagines that the Butter Information Council is somehow like the British Council, or that the World Sugar Research Organization resembles the World Health Organization, should know that these are in part the publicity machines of the butter industry and the sugar industry.

As a rule, the worse a food is for your health, the more money is spent on advertising it. Paid advertising is only one means to promote food. The Food Manufacturers Federation, whose director-general is now Falklands war hero, Sir Jeremy Moore, is formed from a large number of organizations representing the interests of the food industry (notably firms who make highly processed food) and, together with the Food and Drinks Federation, successfully claims to represent the interests of the industry as a whole in Whitehall and Westminster. When Department of Health minister John Patten or Minister of Agriculture Michael Jopling says that the government is looking into ways and means of making food labelling more helpful to the consumer, for instance, they are referring to discussions with the Food Manufacturers Federation and the Food and Drinks Federation (FMF/FDF). Consumers are not represented in these discussions. Nor are Trading Standards Officers whose job it is to enforce the law and so protect the consumer.

Representatives of food manufacturers, and their public relations people, amplify the opinions of individual scientists whose views are helpful to the industry. This is done in a multitude of ways. Food manufacturers pay for some key research into food and health carried out at universities and other places of learning. As one example, research into tooth decay has been funded by Mars Ltd and also by the Cocoa, Chocolate and Confectionery Alliance. Nowadays, university departments of nutrition are supported by the food industry. Senior people who are well known to the public through the media are, often enough, consultants to sections of the food industry concerned to protect the interests of fats, sugars or highly processed starches. And it is common for highly qualified people to move between influential jobs at universities, in industry and in government.

The editor of any major newspaper who carries a feature stating the connection between Western food and Western disease can be sure to receive a substantial number of letters denying that any such connection exists. These letters are usually from manufacturers of unhealthy food and their representatives or advisers but are, quite often, written from private addresses, or else without any reference made to the fact that the writer of the letter has a vested interest. This naughty practice has proved fairly effective in encouraging editors to believe that there are 'two sides' to the food and health story.

16. Yes, But Why is Britain the Backward Nation?

Business will seek to protect its interests the whole world over, and it would be silly to imagine otherwise. And the food giants are just as interested in self-protection in the USA as they are in Britain. So what's the difference?

The difference is: secrecy.

The USA is a society in which it is hard to keep a secret. In matters of public interest, the USA enjoys the Freedom of Information Act. The Senate hearings that led to publication of the McGovern report, for instance, were held in public. The result has proved to be effective consumer groups, and a well-informed press. The doctors who control the American Heart Association, pioneers in the USA in demonstrating that heart disease is caused by eating too much saturated fats, have not kept their views to themselves: the AHA regularly briefs medical correspondents, publishes excellent information in everyday language, devises regular spots on radio, and gives every American citizen the chance to learn the latest about heart disease prevention, by telephoning 1–800 527 4091. This is just one example of the American style of democracy at work.

The UK is a society in which it is easy to keep a secret, especially if it is of public interest. On 14 September 1984, Lord Scarman, Britain's second most senior law Lord, said, 'Parliament, politicians in power, and civil servants have established amongst themselves a tightly knit, secretive system for the efficient creation and fulfilment of consistent nationwide policy. The civil service, as we know it, fits snugly into this cosy system.'

Two days later on 16 September 1984, the *Mail on Sunday*

announced 'doctors studying how Britain's diet is damaging the nation's health are to be asked to sign the Official Secrets Act'. What was the story behind this story? The Committee on Medical Aspects on Food Policy (generally known as COMA; apt, wags say) is a standing committee of scientists who officially advise the Chief Scientist at the Department of Health. Members of this main COMA committee are hand-picked by civil servants in the Department of Health; membership of COMA is, rather like membership of a Royal Commission working party, proof that you have been nominated as one of the elite known as 'the great and the good'.

Members of the main COMA committee have in fact always been required to sign the Official Secrets Act. The new move noted by the *Mail on Sunday* in September 1984, was that the Government decided that members of COMA sub-committees should also be required to sign the Act. Three sub-committees in session in 1985 were on food and the health of infants, schoolchildren and the elderly.

In a leading article, the *Mail on Sunday* roundly stated, 'it remains an extraordinary fact that Britain is the most backward nation in the whole of the Western world, both in the ability of the press properly to investigate "the great and the good", and in the refusal of governments of all complexions actually to trust the people with information to which they are fully entitled.'

Describing this new requirement that COMA sub-committee members sign the Official Secrets Act as 'disgraceful', the *Mail* went on 'if the government decrees that it is an official secret to know about, for example, the incidence of sugar and fat in our daily diet, as it is now saying it is, then what else is being kept from us?'

This is what *The Food Scandal* is all about.

How do COMA committees work? They are activated only when the Department of Health so chooses. For example the national policy on what constitutes a balanced diet is derived from the report of a COMA sub-committee on recommended daily amounts of various 'scheduled' nutrients – protein, vitamins, A, D, B_1, B_2, B_3, C, and calcium, iron and iodine, as well as energy. This list is less than half of the nutrients now well known to be essential to life and health. Many of these are lacking in the highly processed British diet. So why, for example, is there no recommendation for fibre in this report? Nor for four nutrients now well known to be especially important for adolescent and pregnant women, and also lacking in the British diet – vitamins B_6, B_{12}, folic acid and zinc? One reason is that the latest version of the COMA report on recommended daily amounts of nutrients, published in 1981, is basically a reprint of an edition originally published in 1969. The 'balanced diet' as officially laid down by government is in fact unbalanced and inadequate.

No group of scientists has ever publicly queried government control of policy on food and health. The Department of Health, together with the Department of Education and Science, is virtually the monopoly employer of doctors and scientists in Britain, and virtually the monopoly supplier of money for research. Industry supplies most of the rest of the jobs and money and facilities.

Suppose you were a scientist who wanted to investigate the possible causal connection between sugars and heart disease by means of a rigorous study using many people over a long period of time, and using scientific methods designed meticulously to eliminate any kind of bias. The government-backed view is that sugars are not a direct cause of heart disease. A study mounted by the Medical Research Council (funded by the Department of Education and Science) came to this conclusion in 1970, since when there has been a lack of enthusiasm for this area of research. The line, emphasized by the sugar industry, is – don't worry about sugars. So, where would you go for backing, funding, and research facilities?

17. Who, then, Can I Trust?

Trustworthy statements about food and health are made by

people whose knowledge is uncontaminated by political or by commercial considerations.

It must be said that the NACNE report is itself somewhat constrained for political reasons; the scientists on the NACNE committee attempted to produce a report designed both to be scientifically sound and yet politically acceptable.

So far in Britain, the NACNE report, together with the reports published by the Royal College of Physicians on which it in part relies, are as close as we have got to trustworthy committee reports.

With some exceptions, the most reliable individual statements made in Britain about food and health are those by people who were professionally active during the Second World War, when national policy demanded a healthy population; or else by people whose judgement depends on experience in non-Western countries. In either case, many of these people are now past the age of retirement.

18. Is the NACNE Report the Last Word on the Subject?

No, it isn't. It is better seen as the first word on the subject of food and health.

First, the report contains some errors and omissions, which do not affect its thesis. One error, already pointed out (page 12) is the under-estimate of consumption of sugars, and the mistaken view that sugars consumption is dropping, in Britain.

Second, its discussion of fats and protein is too brief. It fails to make a clear distinction between saturated fats and essential fats; and between meat protein (liable to be associated with saturated fats) and vegetable protein (liable to be associated with essential fats). The report overall can be accused of fudging a fundamental issue: the division between whole, fresh food on the one hand, and highly processed food on the other. Anybody can understand that whole, fresh food is liable to be nutritious and that highly processed food is liable not to be nutritious; it is common sense and (as common sense often is) true, too. But committees appointed by the government are vigorously discouraged from pointing an accusing finger at highly processed foods.

Third, the report pays scant attention to minerals and vitamins, mentioning only some of those 'scheduled' by the Department of Health. It also does not query the DHSS recommended daily amounts of these vitamins and minerals. Given that the report relies on British sources (with the one World Health Organization exception) it can be argued that its compilers had no choice; certainly the Department of Health would never have accepted a report which queried the official line. Since in the event the government disowned the report, with hindsight it might as well have been less of a compromise, and made plain that official thinking about vitamins and minerals needs revision.

Fourth, the report has next to nothing to say about the special needs of pregnant and lactating women, and what it has to say about infants, children and adolescents is patchy. There is some virtue in this: reports published by the Department of Health give the impression that the only people who might have any problem about food and health are 'special groups' (like infants, Asian immigrants and elderly people living alone, or pregnant women). The NACNE report makes clear that we all need to change our eating habits. Nevertheless, the importance of positively good food, above all when preparing for pregnancy, is another message vital to the health of the child as well as the mother.

Fifth, cancers are not mentioned as diet-related diseases; this is because no British expert committee has yet reported on diet and cancer. In March 1984 the US government declared that cancers are diet-related diseases and that the first priority with cancers is prevention, after major statements by representative bodies of American doctors. The fact that Western food is a major underlying cause of cancer is not news; the McGovern report made the causal connection six years before NACNE, in

1977. By contrast, in Britain it is still commonly supposed by the general public that the main cause of cancers (apart from smoking and lung cancer) is pollution; but the evidence indicates that Western food is the main single underlying cause of a number of cancers, including cancer of the breast, gullet, stomach, pancreas, colon and rectum.

Sixth, the brief of the report did not extent to food additives, nor food contaminants. This is a major omission: it is estimated that perhaps nine tenths of the food we eat contains colouring, flavouring, preservatives, and other additives; or pesticides, herbicides, traces of hormones, antibiotics, heavy metals, and other contaminants. It has recently been estimated that people in Britain on average eat anything from 6 to 15 lbs of additives per year.

Seventh, the 'interim' or 'short term' goals in the report were added to what turned out to be the penultimate draft in 1983, as a further attempt to make the report acceptable to the Department of Health (and also the Ministry of Agriculture). These cobbled-together goals were added in good faith, but do not have any medical or scientific significance (and were not proposed by the compilers of the report, either); they are there as a compromise. They are small changes that can be made by the individual, by trimming fat from meat, and stopping adding sugar and salt at table, and so forth. They really do not have a proper place in a report setting out national goals for healthy food; proper goals require the collaboration of government and industry.

Eighth, the 'long term' goals in the report, which do have medical and scientific significance, and which are broadly in line with many other similar reports produced over the last ten years or so in various countries, are nevertheless not ideals. Cutting consumption of processed sugars by half is good; best, is cutting out processed sugars altogether. Likewise, cutting consumption of saturated fats in half is good; best, is consuming a diet rich in essential fats and very low in saturated fats. Much the same applies to salt: we need so little sodium compared with what we eat, that effectively the less salt we eat, the better.

The more that is known about food and health, the clearer it becomes that the quality of the food we eat is the key to the quality of our health and therefore our lives. The NACNE report is a beginning, towards that understanding.

19. Now It's Fibre; Before, It Was Vitamins, Protein, then Salads. Isn't This Just the Latest Fashion?

A good question, as they say. We in Britain have learned about nutrition – food and health – in fits and starts.

In the past the British government has been very interested in national nutritional policies. Fifty years ago and more, everybody was taught about 'protective' foods: these were foods that contained specific vitamins (A and D, C, and later B_1, B_2 and B_3). These vitamins were known to protect against deficiency diseases, one of which, rickets (caused by lack of sunlight or of vitamin D) was a scourge of urban children up to the 1930s. Children were issued cod liver oil and halibut liver oil (for vitamin D) and orange concentrate (for vitamin C) during and after the Second World War. And foods were 'fortified' with vitamins: A and D were added to margarine, B_1 and B_3 to white flour and bread, C to fruit drinks, and, later, a variety of vitamins to ready-to-eat breakfast cereals. As a rule, any food advertised as having vitamins added to it, is food which has lost most of its vitamins and minerals while being processed. It is as if a thief takes your purse but then 'fortifies' you by handing you some of the pennies back.

In the 1930s protein was emphasized as of special importance. This is because protein in particular was shown to encourage growth in rats, and at that time doctors believed that millions of British children were suffering or were liable to suffer from malnutrition. The doctors were right to be concerned; but it is probable that millions of children who grew up thin and small in the 1920s and 1930s were suffering from malnutrition in general, not just protein malnutrition. However, experiments with rats showed that a high protein diet caused fast growth and, on this basis, national policy was to grow big bonny bouncing babies on high-protein diets. This is why we still 'believe in' cow's milk, which has a higher protein content than human milk, and why we still think of meat, cheese and eggs as good foods eaten in abundance. Health visitors and dieticians taught old-style still preach the special value of these foods for children.

In the Second World War the government made agricultural self-sufficiency a policy of the highest national priority, and the farming of cows for meat and milk has been vigorously encouraged ever since.

Knowledge gained within the last half-century shows that the high-protein experiment, pursued in Britain and other Western countries with great vigour, has been harmful on a national basis. It is natural for rats and cows to increase in size with great rapidity in early life. By contrast, the natural growth of human bodies is slow; it is the human brain that sets us apart from animals, and the best food for the brain is not protein, but essential fats. (If grandmother told you that fish is good for your brains, she was right.)

Western enthusiasm for protein was an expression of the general enthusiasm for growth – bigger cars, higher salaries, faster expanding gross national products, went with big, tall bodies. Early puberty, also induced by a high-protein diet, was also seen as a Good Thing. But from the social point of view, there is little to be said for young secondary schoolchildren having sex on their minds, nor for pregnant 15-17 year old girls. From the health point of view there is now some evidence from animal experiments that accelerated growth and early sexual maturity lead to faster degeneration in what otherwise would be middle life. The epitaph of the high-protein experiment may prove to be that it bred big beefy people who died young.

Protein is best eaten as food rich in fibre, essential fats, vitamins and minerals, rather than as foods which, like milk, red meat and cheese, are heavy with saturated fats.

After the war, with sweets off the ration, white bread universal, and meat every day regarded as an elementary status symbol, overweight and obesity became more common, and yet slimness became more desirable. Hence the rise of the 'diet' (meaning, of course, the diet regime, the attempt to lose fat) and the 'diet doctor' and the discovery by women's magazines that 'diets' were good for sales. Diet regimes come in all shapes and sizes, and are advertised as being new and different (as well as miraculous etc), but almost all are based on the same principle, which is, eat less: the low calorie principle. The people who devise diet regimes, many of whom should know better, check through lists of analyses prepared by food scientists and select, for their regime, food that is low in calories per a given weight. These foods are often low in calories because of being high in water. The result tends to be food that leaves the body starving.

The tendency now is for people to eat less and less, and get fatter and fatter. This is true of schoolchildren as well as adults. As a nation we need to exercise more, not eat less. The vital importance of regular vigorous exercise throughout life, to stay lean and also healthy, has been largely overlooked in Britain until the early 1980s. Food with lots of water in it is a good choice only when it also contains lots of nourishment. Choose vegetables with substance rather than lettuce; oranges rather than diet cola.

We have been taught to think of food as being basically protein, fat or carbohydrate. These food scientists' distinctions are not helpful in many cases. Meat and cheese are classified as protein foods, yet most of the energy in almost all meat (including 'lean' meat) and in cheese comes from fat. The 'carbohydrate' classification is totally misleading and should be abandoned. Chemically, carbohydrates (monosaccharides, disaccharides and polysaccharides) are similar, and they behave similarly in a test-tube or when burned in a scientist's 'calorimeter' (which measures the energy given off by foods when consumed in a flame). All carbohydrates supply energy (as do protein and fats) and carbohydrates are converted into blood sugar (glucose) when eaten.

As a result, until recently the official tables of food values prepared by scientists lumped the carbohydrate content of foods together. Since carbohydrates supply energy, people who devised low calorie diet regimes looked up the food value tables and lumped together all foods high in carbohydrate as Bad.

Alternatively, food manufacturers whose business is to sell foods high in carbohydrates (processed sugars in particular) spend countless millions of pounds advertising their products as Good. This process continues. So half the time we have been told that bread and potatoes are fattening, and half the time that a Mars a day helps us work, rest and play.

The way out of this confusion is to forget about 'carbohydrate' and think in terms of whole foods (rich in starch) versus highly processed foods (heavy in sugars). It is starchy food in whole form (wholemeal bread, cereals and vegetables) that is the staple food of people relatively free of Western diseases. Sweet food in whole form (fruits, mostly) is also nutritious. On the other hand, processed sugars contain no nourishment, but only calories. It is also true that processed starchy foods (white bread, flour, rice and pastas, for instance) are stripped of much of the fibre, vitamins, minerals and essential fats. Whole starchy food is best; processed sugars are worst.

During the last fifty years the ideas that we have been taught, whether by government, science or industry, whether for reasons of national defence or of commerce, have proved to be outdated or wrong.

Why then should we believe the new message which, in its positive form, is: eat whole fresh food, and prefer food of vegetable origin? This message is based on modern medical and scientific thinking and essentially is contained in dozens of reports now published in Western countries. Perhaps more to the point, it corresponds with eating habits of people throughout history, with the exception of Western countries in the last 150 years. The latest knowledge reflects the oldest wisdom.

20. But Surely Milk is Whole and Fresh?

And, come to that, meat, cheese and butter? You may have noticed advertisements put out by the Butter Information Council saying that we've been enjoying butter for the past ten thousand years. The Milk Marketing Board has in similar terms persuaded Britain, with 20 per cent of the population of the European Community, to drink 40 per cent of the milk produced in the EEC. And here, agribusiness has allies among whole food people representing the Soil Association.

How can food of animal origin – meat, dairy products, milk – be bad for our health?

These foods are not like processed sugars. There is plenty of nourishment in them. The problem is the amount of them we consume, and the amount of saturated fats they contain.

Until the Second World War, most people in Britain on average consumed around 30 per cent of their calories in the form of fats. Now the figure is about 40 per cent. The NACNE report (and the McGovern report) recommends that we reduce the amount of fats we eat to 30 per cent of total calories, the quantity that our grandparents ate.

But what about the Eskimos and the Masai? In their natural habitats the Eskimos eat mostly meat, the Masai warriors drink a lot of cow's milk and blood mixed together, and these people do not suffer from heart disease. So what about that? (You will find that representatives of the Bacon and Meat Manufacturers' Association, the Butter Information Council, and the Milk Marketing Board, are keen on the Eskimo and the Masai.)

First, it is not true that the Eskimos eat only meat, or that

Masai warriors consume only milk and blood. They do when they have to, but when other food is available they eat that, too.

Second, and this is the more important point, the quality of the meat, and the quality of the fat, eaten by people in pre-Westernised societies is altogether different from what we eat. Wild animals, left free to forage on common land and in woodland, are lean; and what fat they have is highly nutritious, being rich in essential fats. By contrast, domesticated animals fed on grass and concentrates become very fat; and this fat is thoroughly unhealthy, being heavy in saturated fats.

Like us, animals are what they eat. And the traditional Eskimo diet, although high in fats, is particularly high in essential polyunsaturated fats because it contains so much fish and seal meat. It is low in saturated fats. We have made our animals unhealthy and when we eat products derived from them we become unhealthy, too.

There is no need to become vegetarian or vegan. Simple changes, such as from full-fat to skimmed milk, and from carcass meat to white and fatty fish (say, half the time) will make quite a difference. Any swap from butter should be to margarine labelled 'high in polyunsaturates'. And try good quality olive oil for cooking. Delicious!

21. Isn't It Just a Question of Eating a Normal Balanced Varied Diet

What is a 'normal balanced varied diet'? The Department of Health definition of a balanced diet, is one which supplies the recommended daily amounts of nutrients it specifies as important for health. These are energy (calories); protein; and nine vitamins and minerals. (Two more vitamins were added in late 1984.) Thus, a school lunch designed to supply one third of the day's nourishment is 'balanced' by being made up of white bread ('fortified' with B vitamins, calcium and iron, as well as containing protein); hard margarine ('fortified' with vitamins A and D); peanut butter or Marmite on the bread (more protein and vitamins); a couple of chocolate biscuits (energy) and a sweet drink ('fortified' with vitamin C on top of its natural vitamin C). So 'balance' is what the Department of Health says is balance. The concept is a survival of the 'food groups' idea still taught to dieticians: balance 'protective' foods (vitamins and minerals) with 'growth' foods (protein) and 'energy' foods (fats and carbohydrates), and you have a 'good' diet.

In this notion of balance there is no thought of fibre; no query about the quality of fats, processed sugars or salt; nothing about a dozen other vitamins and minerals well known to be vital to health; and no need to include any fresh foods at all. As long as the energy level rings the Department of Health bell, any kind of sugar or fat is fine.

This is why the NACNE report states that the current notion of 'balance' in the diet should be abandoned. Like virtue, nobody can object to the idea of balance. Of course 'an unbalanced diet' is a bad idea. It all depends what is meant by 'balance'. The fact is that, over the last 150 years, and more and more within the last thirty years, the British diet has become abnormal, unbalanced, and spuriously varied.

22. Are You Saying (as a Generalization) that the More Highly Processed Food Is, the Worse It Is for Your Health?

Yes.

23. Are All Fats Bad?

No. Some fats are bad; some are positively good for your health. The NACNE report gives the impression that basically fats are bad, and that the paramount issue is that people in Britain should eat less fats. Following this recommendation will in practice do nothing but good to almost all people. But many scientists with special knowledge of fats and health dislike the NACNE attitude to fats, seeing it as unhelpfully negative in certain respects; and the research that continues to surface on the subject does consistently suggest that NACNE needs revision on fats. Here is why.

Eating a lot of saturated fats is bad for health: there's no serious doubt about that. The less saturated fats you eat, the better. However, zero is impossible, because even 'healthy' fats and oils do contain small quantities of saturated fats. The point is that societies whose people are virtually free of heart disease generally eat very small amounts of saturated fats. On the other hand, essential fats are, as their name suggests, vital not only to health, but life itself. The body does not make essential fats; they have to be supplied in the food we eat. (For this reason they are sometimes referred to as 'vitamin F'.) Essential fats are what make polyunsaturated fats positively good for health. (Saturated fats contain no essential fats; like sugars, they are empty calories, or as one authority on the subject calls them, 'trash energy'.)

What is so special about essential fats is that they nourish those parts of the body that are themselves rich in, or largely composed of, essential fats: in particular, the nervous system, the soft part of the spinal column, and the brain.

There is reason to believe that degeneration of these parts of the body can be and is caused by deficiency of essential fats. This area of human health has not yet been thoroughly studied. Meanwhile, birth defects of the brain and spinal column are common in Britain; multiple sclerosis officially remains a mystery disease; and premature senile dementia (middle-aged people who have lost their reason) is an increasing public health worry.

What is certainly true, is that you can't eat too many essential fats when they are a constituent of whole fresh food. If you say good riddance to foods high in saturated fats and processed sugars, you will be able to eat foods like fatty fish, game animals and birds, wholemeal bread, nuts and seeds, all rich in essential fats and many other nutrients, to your stomach's content.

As a nation we consume over four times as much saturated as

polyunsaturated fats. This is a disaster. What has happened is food processing. Saturated fats are stable. They have a long shelf life. With added preservatives, products heavy in saturated fats may have a 'best before' stamp giving a date months after you buy them. They are good for business. The NACNE report recommends that the national average consumption of saturated fats be cut almost in half, to 10 per cent of total calories, but does not recommend that consumption of polyunsaturates be increased from its present level of 4 per cent of calories.

The American McGovern report recommends 10 per cent of calories from saturated fats (the same as NACNE) and a goal of 10 per cent of calories from polyunsaturated fats (radically different from NACNE). The policy of cutting right back on saturated fats, especially in highly processed foods, and at the same time eating plenty of whole foods rich in polyunsaturated fats, is the right policy for good health.

Where should we Britons, an island race, get polyunsaturates from? Everything points to a revival of enthusiasm for fatty fish: herring, mackerel, sprats, kippers and bloaters, and, when you can afford them, trout and salmon. And in addition, game animals and birds: rabbit, hare, venison, pigeon, pheasant, grouse. The tip to follow, is: if you like flesh eat it from creatures that lived and died fit. For tea, for example, kick out the sliced bread and jam, biscuits and cakes, and get back to hunks of wholemeal bread with fish in season: just as delicious, twice as satisfying, and good for you as well.

The war between the 'goody' polyunsaturates and the 'baddy' saturates, reflected in most expert reports on fats, has tended to trample over what may prove to be at least as important an area: the 'neutral' fats, the monounsaturates. Experts who say that good health is all about eating less fats in general have not faced the fact of the olive. The interesting thing about olive oil is that it is low both in saturated and polyunsaturated fats: around three quarters of olive oil is monounsaturated. Now, while people in Britain, Northern

Europe, America and other Western countries eat butter or margarine, people in Mediterranean countries (Greece, Spain, Southern France and Italy, and the Middle East) use olive oil as their staple source of fats. Their rates of suffering and death from fats-related diseases is much lower than in Britain. But – and this is the key point – the amount of fat they consume is often much the same as that consumed in Britain. As an example: Greeks have a longer life expectancy than Britons; the quality of their lives over the age of 60 and 70 (certainly in the countryside) is conspicuously superior; and the rate of death from heart disease in Greece is very much lower than that in Britain. Nevertheless, in terms of calories, Greeks eat as much, or more, calories in the form of fats as people in Britain do – mostly as olive oil. The story in other Mediterranean countries is similar.

What does all this tell us? First, that saturated fats, not fats in general, are the villain. Effectively, this means highly processed foods containing hardened fat, and fatty meat, milk and diary produce. Second, that we do not have to contemplate a gloomy future with no lubrication for our food. In practice, this means sticking to oils high in polyunsaturates like sesame, sunflower, soya, safflower and corn oils, and to olive oil. Third, that good and healthy food doesn't have to leave you hungry. If you take regular vigorous exercise, and use the right oils in food, you can enjoy food without a qualm. There is no need for healthy food to be dry and boring.

24. Are All Sugars Bad?

No. In whole foods (fruits and some vegetables) sugars come associated with fibre, vitamins and minerals, and are absorbed slowly by the body. The same applies to starches in whole foods (bread and potatoes, for instance) which are also slowly absorbed and converted to blood sugar (glucose) in the body.

Processed sugars, on the other hand, are stripped of any

nourishment, and all of them are bad from the health point of view. In addition to their poor nutritional quality, they rot teeth, and lead to abnormal swings in blood sugar level.

The effect of processed sugars on health is probably worse when they are consumed in most concentrated form, as soft drinks, sweets and confectionery, for instance. Highly sugared foods such as ice-cream, biscuits, cakes, pickles, canned fruit, and vegetables, sweetened breakfast cereals, sweetened yoghurts, jams and marmalades, are also bad for health, even though the sugar is more spread out.

When natural sugars from fruits are extracted as juice they too are not altogether desirable: whole fruit is always better.

But generally speaking, sugars from whole foods are fine; otherwise, always seek to avoid sugars. Look at the label. Look for products labelled 'sugar-free', there are more of them now.

25. How Good Is the Evidence Against Salt?

The salt we eat is made up of two essential nutrients: the minerals sodium and chlorine (as sodium chloride, or NaCl in scientific terms). It is therefore strictly nonsense to propose that salt is bad: we need salt to live. The question is, do we consume too much salt, and, if so, what are the consequences?

Shortly after the NACNE report was published, another report, 'Dietary Salt and Health', was reaching an advanced stage of preparation. This report on salt was being prepared by the Faculty of Community Medicine, the professional body for doctors concerned with public health, associated with the Royal College of Physicians in London.

In the draft preface of the report Professor Alwyn Smith, President of the Faculty, wrote:

> The rationale for reducing dietary intake of salt centres around the importance of preventing and controlling raised blood pressure, which is a major cause of heart disease and stroke. Hypertension has now reached epidemic proportions – equal in scale to the

serious infectious diseases of the last century like tuberculosis, cholera and smallpox . . . There is an urgent need not only to accept that we probably eat too much salt for our good but also to take action to lower dietary intake.

The salt report is about the same length as the entire NACNE report. Some of the more memorable points in the salt report are a quotation from Huang Ti, 'if too much salt is used in food the pulse hardens', written in 2300 BC; the fact that average British intake of salt is 10–20 times more than the body needs; and the additional fact that only 7 per cent of salt produced in Britain is used in food. The report also points out that excess salt consumption is linked with stomach cancer as well as high blood pressure (hypertension) and stroke.

The report confirmed the long-term NACNE goal and called for a halving of national salt intake, and a goal of 5 grams a day. This means a goal of 2 grams of sodium a day: almost all the salt we consume is in the form of ordinary cooking or 'table' salt, NaCl, which is formed from 40 per cent sodium (Na) and 60 per cent chloride (Cl), and is added to our food in manufacture, as well as in the home.

As this new edition of *The Food Scandal* went to press, 'Dietary Salt and Health' still had not been published. This time the hold-up has not been caused by government and industry, but by the medical profession itself, or, more specifically, by those doctors who are saying that there is no good evidence to link salt and high blood pressure.

The salt report was circulated in draft in 1984 for comments and criticism from interested parties. One result was a long letter from 13 doctors published in *The Lancet* of 25 August 1984. In a veiled attack on the salt report (still not published, remember) the 13 doctors wrote:

The usual and scientific standards for weighing evidence and giving advice . . . seem to have been forgotten in an evangelical crusade to present a simplistic view of the evidence which will prove attractive to the media.

The letter to *The Lancet* ended by asking for massive funding for studies of the national diet.

The next day the *Sunday Express* published an editorial stating that advice to reduce salt intake was evidently 'utter twaddle' and that before doctors 'next try to scare the nation out of its wits they actually bother to find out what they are talking about..'

What is the argument all about?

Nobody seriously disputes that salt may well be connected with high blood pressure; in a later letter to *The Lancet* (8 December) the dissenting doctors agreed that the proposals that 'hypertension may be induced by excessive dietary salt intake and that it may be prevented or moderated by salt restriction are plausible, important and susceptible to evaluation'. But (they said) the evidence is not strong enough; only some of the population may be adversely affected by salt; and experiments have sometimes shown that salt reduction does not help high blood pressure. If in doubt, they suggest, do nothing. 'A heavy responsibility rests on those who would make dietary recommendations to whole unsupervised populations, without good evidence.' You have of course come across these arguments before; they are much the same as the arguments against the NACNE report.

One great virtue of NACNE in general and 'Dietary Salt and Health' in particular, is that nobody has ever seriously suggested that people in normal health will come to any harm if they consume less salt (and saturated fats, processed sugars and alcohol). On the other hand, drugs used to treat diet-related diseases can and frequently do cause harm. The case against the Western diet in general is so strong that the burden of proof lies with those who assert that it is not a public health problem.

Is salt harmful to the health of everybody, in the quantity now consumed in Britain? Probably not. Likewise, it is pretty certain that only a fraction of the population is vulnerable (or sensitive) to high levels of saturated fats and processed sugars in the diet. But there is no reason to believe that the same fraction of the population is sensitive to salt, saturated fats and processed sugars. It is prudent to act upon the assumption that if one harmful element in the diet doesn't get you, another one may. If any element of the diet is consumed vastly in excess of what the human body has evolved to handle it is common sense to suspect it; and consumption of salt in Britain is excessive.

Some studies have indeed shown that when people with blood pressure are put on low-salt diets, their blood pressure does not change much, if at all. Other studies do show a beneficial lowering of blood pressure. In Belgium a national campaign reduced daily salt consumption from 15 grams to 9 grams a day between 1968 and 1981 and, in this period, there was a drop in deaths from stroke and stomach cancer.

However, in some people, high blood pressure may be irreversible. Similarly, some people with diseased arteries may not be successfully treated by a diet low in saturated fats, because it may be too late for them. But even if the only result of a low-salt diet was no increase in blood pressure, this would be of benefit to people who suffer from high blood pressure, because the problem becomes worse with age.

In any case, to say that a low-salt diet may not be successful treatment for high blood pressure is one thing. To say that a high-salt diet is an important cause of high blood pressure is a different thing. If you pour ink on clothes, they become stained. The stain does not go away if you stop pouring the ink.

There is no real doubt that salt is a major public health problem. There is, however, considerable doubt about exactly what it is about salt that is causing the problem.

Sodium, chlorine (as chloride) and potassium, work together in the body, to balance the fluid content in and outside the cells of the body. A high salt intake is also a high chloride intake, and some experts think that excess chloride as well as or even instead of high sodium, may be the problem.

A high salt intake is likely in practice to mean low potassium intake. Fresh vegetables and fruit are high in potassium, but, when processed, usually have added salt. For instance, potatoes are high in potassium and low in sodium, whereas potato crisps are low in potassium, high in salt. There again, home-made soup, reflecting the value of the vegetables it is made from, is high in potassium, low in sodium (unless salt is added); whereas canned soups are very high in salt. One can of soup can contain very nearly 1 gram of sodium, or 2·5 grams of salt.

Modern thinking is that we should consume more potassium than sodium: half as much again. In fact, we in Britain on average consume twice as much sodium as potassium. It may be that high blood pressure is caused by too much sodium, too much chloride, not enough potassium, or some combination. This is an important medical issue, and a major World Health Organization study, Intersalt, due to report in 1986, will study 10,000 people aged between 20 and 59 in 50 centres all over the world to examine these different hypotheses. In the words of Professor Jeremiah Stamler, leader of the project, Intersalt should provide 'the strongest body of evidence ever assembled' on the subject.

While the scientists are sorting this one out, the practical advice remains the same: eat plenty of fresh vegetables (for potassium); cut out highly processed food (and thus sodium and chloride); and get used to food that tastes of itself rather than salt.

Some publicity has been given to the view that lack of calcium contributes to high blood pressure. The source of this story was a public symposium held in the USA, sponsored by Campbell's Soups. Moreover, according to *Nutrition Action*, the magazine published for consumers in the USA by the Center for Science in the Public Interest, Dr David McCarron, the doubtless sincere champion of the calcium idea, receives financial support from the US National Dairy Council. (Milk is a major source of calcium, none of which is lost in skimmed milk.)

In America, Campbell's soups have been in legal difficulties. The Consumer Frauds division of the office of the Attorney General of New York accused Campbells in 1984 of misleading the 'consumers into believing that eating Campbell's soup promotes good health, when in fact a single serving of the soup contains more salt than is recommended for an entire day's intake'. Campbells withdrew their 'soup is healthy food' campaign and paid $25,000 costs. (Campbell's soups are no more salty than other canned soups.) The evidence against salt is good enough. It will be strengthened when and if 'Dietary Salt and Health' is published.

26. Is the Message That We Should Eat More Fibre the Same as the 'F-Plan'?

Not really, no. It is worth mentioning Audrey Eyton's *F-Plan Diet* because of its staggering commercial success: the book has sold over two million copies in Britain, spin-offs have spun off, and it's a fair bet that any reader of this book has looked at Mrs Eyton's book.

The F-Plan recommends fibre, and Mrs Eyton says that she is against fats, sugars and salt. In practice, though, her book emphasizes fibre to an unpalatable extent, and also recommends bran supplements. And many of her simple recipes are heavy in fats, sugars and/or salt.

In any case, the F-Plan is not a plan for healthy eating so much as a plan for dieting, by means of reducing calories. The special ingredient in the F-Plan is fibre—lots of it—which, Mrs Eyton claims, is a slimming agent. There is a little something in this claim, but not much. The way to become slim and stay slim is not calorie-cutting, but healthy food and exercise.

27. Isn't This Just What the Health Food Enthusiasts Have Been Saying All Along?

Up to a considerable point, yes. In previous generations a line of doctors not only preached the value of whole food, and prescribed it, but also manufactured it. Dr Thomas Allinson baked a special wholemeal loaf. He was therefore barred from practising as a doctor. The Allinson bread now on sale is wholemeal but has additives in it. Dr John Kellogg developed corn flakes for his patients at the Battle Creek sanitorium in Michigan. His brother Will (the W. K. Kellogg) added sugar to the recipe to make the early version of corn flakes as we now know them. Dr W. O. Bircher-Benner found that raw fruit had restorative powers and invented muesli, from fresh fruit with whole cereal. Muesli is now marketed as mostly cereal with dried fruit, and usually with lots of sugars too.

In Britain the whole food movement has been greatly influenced by another line of doctors in this century, from Sir Robert McCarrison to Surgeon-Captain T. L. Cleave, and now Dr Hugh Sinclair, Dr Denis Burkitt and Dr Hugh Trowell. They have proved to have a profound effect on modern medical and scientific thinking.

Unfortunately, though, some 'health food' writers and enthusiasts have tended to give healthy food rather a bad name. Recipes often include wholemeal flour and no white sugars, which is fine. But a lot of the food is dull and boring; and uses masses of fats and brown sugars or honey, which is bad. Moreover, some *whole food* shops, often run as co-operatives, sell basic whole food commodities in bulk. They are often cheap, and may stock other fresh, good quality foods. There are many *health food* shops which stock good, healthy food but some overstress vitamin and mineral supplements in the form of pills, which are very profitable, and in this way can distract customers from whole food.

If you know where to shop, and if you are prepared to read labels and ask questions of shopkeepers, you can buy whole, healthy food in the typical supermarket, greengrocer and fishmonger as easily as you can in the typical 'health food' shop. You do need to know what to look for. That is what this book is all about.

Some healthy food is 'health food', and some 'health food' is healthy. But the health food trade is a business, like any other.

In the USA very many supermarkets now have healthy food sections and shelves where you can buy food free of sugars and salt. (These counters are not usually labelled 'healthy food', for obvious reasons – what would the customers then think of what was on sale elsewhere!) Leading British retailers, notably Tesco, are now taking initiatives and (no doubt to the disgust and chagrin of some manufacturers) improving the information on 'own-label' products, including details of fats, sugars and salt. Encourage this trend.

28. Can Food Cure Disease?

Disease can be prevented, checked, relieved or cured. 'Cure' means complete recovery of good health, after disease. You can't be cured without having a disease in the first place.

Very often, people take their good health for granted and neglect themselves until illness or disease takes hold; and many of these diseases now common in Britain do not show themselves until after years or even decades of undetected development. These 'degenerative' diseases often do not show themselves until middle or late age: but they come on in earlier life.

Degenerative diseases are usually diet-related to a greater or lesser extent, but it is, alas, futile to suppose that any treatment is certain to cure them. Many sufferers, disappointed with conventional medical treatment, turn to 'alternative' or 'fringe' medicine often as a last resort. Some of these 'fringe' practitioners are pedlars of false hopes.

Arthritis sufferers seem to be a special target. Advertisements that appear in the health press aimed at arthritis sufferers may advocate multivitamins, or Korean Ginseng, or kelp tablets, or even colonic irrigation.

Such claims sound much like those of the Victorian snake oil salesmen. Some outer regions of the 'health food' trade have a dubious reputation. Notice, though, that the hope held out is of relief, not cure; and also that the treatment is usually not provided with whole food, but with supplements or pills or potions used as medicine.

The most important benefit of good food is not that it cures disease, but that it prevents disease and promotes good health. And no individual person can ever know that he or she did not develop arthritis, or heart disease, or cancer, because of eating good food. This is one reason why a lot of people are sceptical about the value of good food; for everybody likes to believe that disease is something that happens to the other person.

But what when disease develops? Good food cannot do harm in any circumstances (apart from some rare disorders, harped on, illogically, by the 'food is irrelevant' medical brigade). If good food has any effect, in practically all circumstances it can only be to improve health.

Just what the effect of good food will be, depends on the disease. Take two diseases caused by bad food. Constipation is principally caused by lack of cereal fibre in the diet. Time and again doctors in hospitals have shown that constipation is cured by a high fibre diet. Tooth decay is principally caused by processed sugars. But once decay has penetrated the tooth enamel it can only be treated, not cured. In the early stages of decay teeth can re-mineralize, but usually the value of cutting out sugars is confined to the prevention of future tooth decay.

What about heart disease? It is practically certain that heart disease cannot be cured by good food. It is almost equally certain that the development of heart disease is slowed and perhaps arrested by a diet rich in whole, fresh food; and experiments with animals suggest that a diet that all but eliminates saturated fats in favour of polyunsaturated fats may reverse the atherosclerotic process. Regular vigorous exercise may have the same effect. But anybody who supposes that good food can cure advanced heart disease misunderstands the nature of the disease which, when advanced, begins to destroy the fabric of the arterial wall.

The reason why, despite uncertainty about the exact benefits of good food, and individual variability of response, knowledgeable doctors can recommend good food to people with heart disease without hesitation, is because good food cannot do harm. The same cannot be said of drugs used to relieve the symptoms of heart disease, which often have alarming adverse effects.

Some distinguished doctors, notably Alec Forbes and Jan de Winter in Britain, are committed to the view that diet is vital not only to prevent cancers of all types, but also in their treatment. But so often, alas, cancer sufferers turn to alternative therapies – dubious or, in the case of Dr Forbes and Dr de Winter, admirable – too late for hope of cure. Cancer is a strange disease. Advanced cancers can sometimes retreat, and a virulent cancer may disappear. Good food can only support any such process; but it is not a 'magic bullet'.

Any disease that causes destruction of the fabric of the body eventually cannot be cured by any means – drugs, surgery, or food. Nevertheless, it may be that some diseases now regarded as intractable are not only at least in part caused by the typical British diet, but are also treatable, even if not curable, by good food.

Doctors will continue to argue about whether or not specific diseases are diet-related, and whether or not they can be successfully treated by good food. Meanwhile you can, with complete confidence, cut out the empty calories in favour of the nourishment in whole, fresh food. The diet that is the best protection against disease is also the diet that will be of most benefit to people who suffer from disease. And the story is the same for practically all diseases. Advice about an anti-diabetes diet, as distinct from an anti-cancer or anti-heart disease or anti-obesity diet, can be misleading and confusing. For whether you are concerned about disease, or about positive good health, the story is the same: whole fresh food is not a magic cure, nothing is; but it will strengthen you.

29. What Is 'The Food Scandal'?

Why are the rates of premature death from heart disease in
Britain now the highest in the world? Why are the rates of
death from heart disease falling in many other countries but not
significantly in Britain? Why are the rates of premature death
from all causes now higher in Britain than in other EEC
countries and in Scandinavia, and highest of all in Scotland,
Northern Ireland and Wales? Why is premature death so
strongly class-related, with so many of the poor suffering and
dying many years before their natural time?

An adjournment debate on the subject of prevention of heart
disease was held in the House of Commons on 16 July 1984.
Conservative MP Jonathan Aitken said 'the prevention of heart
disease is a most important health issue which, until recently,
has been tragically neglected by public opinion, by large parts
of the food industry, and by the government departments that
should be most interested in it'.

He went on to say 'one need only consider some international
comparisons to understand that there seems to be a peculiar, if
not downright sinister, local dimension to the heart disease
problem, which makes Britain the heart attack capital of the
world'. Why has government evidently been inert, faced with
the evidence that heart disease is preventable? 'The recent best-
selling book, *The Food Scandal*, by Caroline Walker and
Geoffrey Cannon is, as the title suggests, an attack on what the
authors consider to be officialdom's scandalous reluctance to
implement the recommendations of NACNE and other such
reports,' said Jonathan Aitken.

Aitken's own contribution to the national debate goes to
show that food and health is not a party political issue. Indeed,
the previous Labour government failed to take any initiative.
The Department of Health publication *Prevention and Health:
Everybody's Business* was issued as a 'consultative document'
when Barbara Castle was in charge at the DHSS, in 1977. The
phrase, 'consultative document' has a familiar ring; like

'discussion paper', used in the title of the NACNE report as issued by the Health Education Council, 'consultative document' is a way of saying 'we may not mean anything that's within'.

But did the Labour government have anything disturbing to say about the prevention of heart disease in 1977, the year of the McGovern report in the USA? No, it did not. 'To the extent, therefore that coronary heart disease is determined by a man's lifestyle' the consultative document said (what about women?) 'the prime responsibility for his own health falls on the individual'.

In other words, if you are a greedy or lazy silly billy, and get heart disease, it's your fault for not going to the public library and reading it up in *The Lancet*. This view is also known as 'blaming the victim'.

And what did the Labour government have to say about sugars and tooth decay? 'A childhood without sweets may well be regarded by many as a fate worse than an adult without teeth.' Lines like this, drafted by civil servants for the approval of politicians, help to explain why the DHSS is sometimes referred to as the Department of Stealth and Total Obscurity.

The Labour party in opposition in 1985 has, in part thanks to the initiative of Dr Jeremy Bray, now remembered that food and health is a political issue. And there are signs that the other political parties are waking up. Whether action of real significance will be taken by the Conservative Government in power in 1985, is another matter.

There is nothing new in the proposal that food and health is a political issue. Fifty years ago, speaking to government, John Boyd Orr said, in his classic study 'Food, Health and Income', 'from the point of view of the state, the adoption of a standard of diet lower than the optimum is uneconomic. It leads to a great amount of preventable disease and ill-health which lay a heavy financial burden on the State . . . it is probable that an enquiry would show that the cost of bringing a diet adequate for health within the purchasing power of the poorest would be less than treating the disease and ill-health that would thereby be prevented.' Some time within the last half century, Boyd Orr's words, as relevant now as then, were forgotten.

As Jonathan Aitken stated, the 'scandal' in the title of this book refers specifically to the unconscionable delays in publication of the NACNE report. But the NACNE story is only one passage in a volume of scandal. The NACNE delays were but two years in a whole decade of deliberate refusal by public servants to listen to what their medical advisers were saying, or to find out for themselves what anybody with a proper sense of public responsibility could have determined, if only from conversations with Americans.

The 1984 COMA report, *Diet and Cardiovascular Disease*, is well known. But there was another COMA report, *Diet and Coronary Heart Disease* in 1974. 'The panel has taken three years and ten drafts to produce their report' wrote Sir George Godber, then chief scientist at the Department of Health, in the preface. What did the 1974 COMA report recommend? One member of the panel, Professor John Yudkin, stated his view that sugars rather than fats are to blame for heart disease. But the panel's recommendation, from the other eleven members, was 'the amount of fat in the United Kingdom diet, especially saturated fats from both animal and plant sources, should be reduced'.

What happened between 1974 and 1981, when the NACNE sub-committee under Professor James was set up? Words without action. What happened between 1981 and 1983, and the publication of the NACNE report? Nothing. What happened between 1983 and the 1984 publication of the second COMA report? A media hullabulloo, but government was 'waiting for COMA'. If action had been taken in these ten wasted years, as it was in America, how many people could have been saved from death by heart disease alone? Hundreds of thousands. What does the word 'scandal' mean? 'A grossly discreditable circumstance, event or condition of things'.

Should this book be called *The Food Scandal*? If nothing happens now, the word will be too mild.

30. What Are the Chances of the British People, as a Whole, Eating Healthy Food?

For the last hundred years and more, government has accepted a responsibility to ensure that the food supply is safe and clean. Nearly fifty years ago, government accepted further responsibility, for a healthy food supply, and maintained this responsibility until after the last World War. Until government once again accepts that health is as central to public health policy as is an uncontaminated water supply, death registers will remain dominated by diet-related diseases.

You, reading this book, may well be able to change your eating habits for the better, today, or at least after your next shopping expedition. Indeed, *The Food Scandal* is written with the purpose not only of outlining the message of the NACNE report in plain English, but also of enabling any individual to eat well.

But are you free to choose good food? If you are one of a middle-class adult couple living in a city, prepared to read books and labels and cross-question shop assistants and managers, the answer is almost certainly yes.

But if you have a child at school, a partner dependent on canteen food, or a member of your family in hospital, it's a different story. Yes, you can take the line of most resistance and supply wholemeal sandwiches and fruit (say) from home. But what if you live in a small country town whose 'general store' has only tired brown bread and oranges to offer? Yes, you can bake your own bread and dig up the lawn in any garden you may have and plant vegetables and fruit. But should healthy food be hard to find?

The idea that we are all free as individuals to choose healthy food was until 1985 embraced by the Labour Party as well as the Conservatives. It is an idea that makes incomplete sense for the unemployed, manual workers, farm labourers, children in large families, single-parent families, pensioners, students, young couples, and most people in other low-income groups, including ethnic minorities.

Freedom of choice depends on the ability to choose, and knowledge of what the choices are. We are not free to choose to buy and eat good food unless we have the money to pay for it, unless it is made available to us, and unless we know the difference between good and bad food. And the fact is that millions of British people either cannot afford healthy food, or else cannot find it in their neighbourhood; and in any case have been gulled into the belief that highly processed food is all they need.

People in industry are not public servants. Business is business, and directors of companies are responsible to their board and shareholders, whether the business is telecommunications or tea, banking or boil-in-a-bag beef, offshore oil or inshore fats, circuses or bread.

The quality of the food grown, bred, made and sold in Britain will change for the better only after we, the citizens who eat it, demand change. That process is now happening. Only then will a political party capable of forming a government decide that healthy food could be a campaign issue. That process is also now happening.

It would be wrong to assume that, once they are fully informed, farmers and the food industry will resist change. Until now they have been the victims of conflicting messages, just like the rest of us. When the recommendations of the McGovern Committee were announced in 1977, Robert Dole, Republican Senator for Kansas, a farming state, was interviewed, and asked what his voters should think of his support for the McGovern recommendations. He said, first, that farmers did not want to die prematurely from heart attacks; and, second, that American agriculture and industry had made the country great by responding to change. The same is true of Britain.

People in government are public servants. It is the responsibility of the politicians and civil servants in the Department of Health, the Ministry of Agriculture, and other government departments to see to it now that the food we eat is healthy as well as safe and clean. In the 1930s government insisted on a national plan for healthy food for a practical reason: young men had to be made fit to fight a war. In the 1980s there is a new equally practical reason: unless the national food supply is healthy, sooner or later the National Health Service will collapse under the weight of patients being referred with (often undiagnosed) diet-related diseases. And a bankrupt NHS means a bankrupt State.

The last word is with Boyd Orr, writing in 1936. 'It remains, however, to adjust our food policy so that the great wealth of food which we have or can produce will be brought within the purchasing power of the poorest. This is no easy task. It will require economic statesmanship of the highest order. But in a democratic country the necessary legislation must be preceded by an intelligent demand on the part of the people.'

PART III

Your Food and Your Health: What To Do

THE GREAT BRITISH DIET. THE MYTH OF MRS BEETON.
THE COLLISION BETWEEN HEALTH AND WEALTH.

So much for theory and science. Where does it leave you, the shopper, cook and consumer of three meals a day, 1,095 meals a year?

The quality of the food we eat and drink is vital and fundamental. If we eat good food, we give ourselves the best chance of enjoying good health. If we eat bad food, we will suffer, certainly in the long term. But food is not just a physical matter. It provides entertainment, hospitality, warmth, fun and pleasure. Can we enjoy healthy food? Can meals containing less saturated fats, sugars and salt ever be fun? And won't the resulting food be a bit un-British?

Dare to suggest to many British citizens that it would be healthier to eat less fats and sugars, and you might get a good ticking off for trying to ruin British food and culture. Take your peculiar foreign ideas to the funny food shop round the corner that sells beans and prunes in sacks. Cream cakes are British and won't be budged. And so are chocolate, and biscuits, roast beef, butter, sponge cake, hamburgers, fish and chips, liquorice all-sorts, ice cream and doughnuts. Food with less fats and sugars wouldn't just be un-British, it would also be no fun to eat, not the kind of stuff you could offer your friends for dinner. And on the level of economics, eating less fats and sugars would ruin the farmers' livelihood and break the back of the British food industry.

The British public is defensive about its national eating habits. Yet the food we eat today has little to do with the food we ate 150 years ago, or even in the 1950s. Pasta, noodles, yoghurt, hamburgers, muesli, Camembert cheese, roasted peanuts, aubergines, peppers, satsumas, garlic sausage – none of these is British in origin and all of them have been introduced recently. Far from being resistant to change, the British public is remarkably adaptable to new foods. Take a look in your own fridge or larder and see how many 'foreign' foods you use daily.

The Great British Diet

In the last twenty to thirty years, Cypriot, Chinese, Indian, Pakistani, American and Italian restaurants and take-aways have been springing up all over the place. Sweet and sour pork is a national favourite. Footballers take pride in sweating their way through platefuls of vindaloo. Did you think that Colonel Sanders served in the Royal Fusiliers, or that the Macdonald of the hamburgers hails from the Highlands, or that the Pizza Express was the London to Carlisle mail train?

Foreign foods and foreign ways of cooking them are extremely popular. Foods which were exotic and unknown a generation ago are now commonplace. We have to thank our resident ethnic minorities and foreign travel for many new and healthy foods such as pasta, rice, yoghurt, peppers, pizza. At the same time some introductions have been less beneficial – hamburgers, crisps in all shapes, sizes and flavours, and cream cakes.

Until very recently, the average British diet was a pretty

miserable affair. The common people's food in the nineteenth century consisted chiefly of bread and potatoes, supplemented with very small amounts of fat and meat. Milk, butter, cheese, fresh fruit and vegetables were luxuries few could afford. Sugar was taxed until 1874.

The Myth of Mrs Beeton

In 1861 Mrs Beeton produced her first cookery book. Writing for a newly emerging middle class, she demonstrated how they could make use of the increasing quantities of meat, fats and sugar at their disposal. Embodying what we now think of as traditional British food, Mrs Beeton's methods, and those of 'ghost-writers' who rewrote her book after her death to incorporate more and more gross recipes, became classic. She has recently been updated by Jane Grigson in an *Observer* series on British food, which was subsidized with £350,000 from the food industry. The new Beeton-style cooks and their families dined on excessive fats, sugars and meat. They suffered from gout, died of strokes and 'seizures' and of many other illnesses that they did not associate with their food.

Around a hundred years ago, sugar became dirt cheap, and the British 'sweet tooth' was bred. But the culinary habits of the middle classes were still restricted to a minority. Since that time, cookery books and women's magazines have overflowed with Beeton-style recipes, which we now think of as the 'natural' British diet. It consists of food regularly eaten by all classes only in the last forty years.

The idea of a 'traditional' British (Beeton-style) food is to all intents and purposes a myth. The modern Western diet is an historical aberration, eaten only by a minority in Victorian days, and by the majority of us only in the last two generations.

In the bad old Victorian days, the mass of the population was underfed, underweight, and short of protein, vitamins and minerals. In the 1980s, the mass of the population is also in a bad way. We eat 100 lb of sugars and 100 lb of fats a year. Two thirds of the energy in our food comes from fats, sugars and alcohol. Over three quarters of our food is processed, poor in or even empty of minerals, vitamins, essential fats and fibre. Many of the convenience foods we eat have added chemicals whose long-term effects are unknown and cumulative. Add to that the known dangers of cigarettes and industrial pollution, and we are clearly in trouble.

The Collision Between Wealth and Health

Agriculture and food-processing are big business. The best food commodities are those that 'keep'. Sugars are the best commodity of all: they are concentrated, pure, cheap, do not rot, very palatable, uniform, and easy to make, pack and transport. Tate & Lyle, who retain the monopoly on sucrose imported into Britain, announced a turnover of £1,722 million in 1984, and a record increase in profits to £69·2 million.

Processed sugar in its various forms now finds its way into the majority of packaged foods on the supermarket shelves. The food industry likes it because it is a relatively cheap, stable bulking agent. Mixed with fats, flour, colouring, flavouring and preservatives, it produces an enormous range of products – biscuits, cakes, instant puddings. It even finds its way into savoury foods. Ours is a sweet and sickly diet.

The most unhealthy fats are those that are most profitable. Useful, essential fats are found in vegetable seed oils, nuts, fresh green vegetables, fruits, and fresh fish, and meat from animals reared in traditional ways. But they are usually unstable, prone to rancidity and are therefore not popular in food processing. Unhealthy fats, on the other hand, are those that tend to be solid and stable at room temperature. The food manufacturer selects ingredients which will travel well and cheaply and not give rise to complaints.

Salt is used as a preservative. Once very expensive, it was our only means of keeping meats and vegetables over the winter months. Without it, many would undoubtedly have died. Salt is still added to food to preserve it. Cheese and bacon are obvious examples. But our taste for it lingers on despite the introduction of alternative methods of preservation such as accelerated drying and freezing.

In addition to the benefits to food processors of stable but unhealthy ingredients such as saturated fats, sugars and salt, there is the newer problem brought about by technology: the invention of chemical food additives. The problems facing those concerned about the health of the nation today are very similar to those confronting their nineteenth-century forebears who tried to deal with adulteration of food by dirt and cheap substitutes. Our shops abound with products whose main ingredients are saturated fats, sugars, salts, highly processed starches, artificial colouring, flavouring and preservatives. Not a piece of fruit or vegetable in the recipe, no meat, no fish.

These foods contain ingredients whose presence is listed on the wrapper (although many additives, improvers, bleaches and other chemicals permitted in foods do not have to be declared), yet we do not know the quantities present. Is the manufacturer of a 'chicken flavoured' crisp containing no chicken whatever any less guilty of adulteration than the nineteenth-century manufacturers of 'tea' containing tea dust or no tea at all? The contamination of our food with sugars, fats and artificial additives is institutionalized in a long list of rules proposed by the Ministry of Agriculture, Fisheries and Food, and legalized by Parliament. These regulations do not satisfy the health of the nation. They are put there for the convenience of the manufacturers, among whom there are some whose sole intention it is to make more from less, to turn cheap ingredients into expensive products.

The fundamental truth about food is that there is a collision between what is currently good for business and what is good for health. Potatoes eaten as potatoes are healthy and cheap. Potatoes turned into crunchy snacks are unhealthy and expensive. Yet it makes economic sense to turn more and more potatoes into such products before we buy them, because the processing uses machinery, technology, advertising, packaging and people. This principle underlies the profitability of huge sections of the food industry.

There is the added problem of direct government intervention to support certain interests. The EEC abounds with mountains of butter, dried milk, meat, vegetables, fruit, wine and sugar, brought about by an absurd system of subsidies that encourages production of foods in quantities we cannot eat. These interventions are outside the control of consumers. The theory that 'supply satisfies demand' is quite clearly wrong. Instead, governments introduce subsidies to encourage children to drink fatty milk at school, to encourage us to buy butter instead of margarine. The EEC has a ludicrous set of schemes to reduce these mountains to hillocks. We pay for it.

Amid this unhealthy state of affairs, there is a welcome move by some of the leading supermarkets and food manufacturers in Britain to make their products more healthy. We should give them our support. Food containing less saturated fats, sugars and salt should be imaginatively prepared, delicious to eat. With all that food technology can now offer us, there are more opportunities for food manufacturers to provide us with healthy foods that taste good and are easy to prepare.

Supermarkets, greengrocers and fishmongers all sell good food, but you have to know how to pick and choose. The next part of this book tells you what to look for. For the first time in British history, the mass of the British population could have access to clean, healthy, varied and delicious food in sufficient quantity for all. Agriculture and industry, and consumers demanding more healthy products, should work together towards this national goal. Our survival in good health is what this book is all about. It is a policy for long life.

CHAPTER 1

Butter, Margarine, Fats and Oils

FATS VERSUS OILS. SATURATED, POLYUNSATURATED, AND
ESSENTIAL FATS. THE HORRORS OF HYDROGENATION.
CHOLESTEROL IN FOODS.

The public has little awareness of the ingredients of fats and
oils. So says *Mintel*, a market intelligence publication which
often reports on the food market in Britain. Its observation is
hardly surprising, for when did you last walk into a supermarket and find a tub of margarine or a bottle of oil carrying a
nice big label telling you exactly which fats and oils it contains,
and in what quantities? And how much polyunsaturated fats,
and anyway what does that mean?

The answer is, of course, hardly ever. British manufacturers
are not required by law to give you this information. But without it, how can you know which foods are the most healthy to
eat?

In a society that increasingly relies on processed foods, the
amount and quality of fats we eat every day becomes more and
more obscure. In the old days of bread and dripping, fat was
fat. It was either butter (if you could afford it), or lard, or
dripping, or a little bacon fat. Margarines did not appear until
the second half of the nineteenth century. The mass of the
population ate very few foods: bread, potatoes, oats, a little

treacle or sugar, very little meat, hardly any milk and cheese, a few root vegetables, greens if available and cheap enough, and a little fat. Biscuits, cakes, breakfast cereals, crisps, canned meats – these things did not begin to have a real impact until this century. 'British food' is always changing.

Historically, most British people have eaten fat sparingly. Only the rich could afford it; most people were poor. Increasing affluence and the development of food technology have resulted in a supply of fatty foods undreamt of 100 years ago. Mars Bars, Monster-Munch, Skull Crushers, chocolate chip cookies, hamburgers, dream-topping, filled wafer biscuits; for many people these are now everyday foods. We eat them, but we have little idea of what they contain.

The nation has steadily consumed an increasingly processed and fatty diet, more oils, more margarines, more processed fats. Our food now provides the perfect fatty mixture for the development of clogged-up arteries. We have the highest rate of heart disease in the world, and our daily food is the underlying cause.

Until the government and the food industry make a positive effort to solve this social problem by encouraging the production of more healthy food, unfortunately it remains an individual problem for each one of us. For without a public health programme to encourage better cooking in hospitals, canteens and restaurants, without warning labels on unhealthy foods and more incentives for agriculture and the food manufacturers to produce healthy ones, we have to rely on our own warning signals. We need to travel round the shops with a guidebook. Much of our food should be avoided at all cost because of its harmful fats. We need to know what our food contains, and the labels on food should give us this information.

The Sock Problem

Why on earth should we be so ignorant about our food? How does it happen that we do not know precisely what has gone into a tin of baked beans, a loaf of bread, or a tub of margarine? The label is required by law simply to give you a list of ingredients in descending order of quantity. It does not tell you the exact amount of fats, or sugars, or salt, or indeed of any of the ingredients. Some manufacturers voluntarily supply this information, but as a rule they are not required to do so by law.

If you go shopping to buy a pair of socks, you will find that socks are labelled. The label tells you what the socks are made of; it tells you how much of each fibre there is. It even tells you where the socks were made, and how to wash them. Socks, 80 per cent cotton, 20 per cent nylon. Made in Hong Kong. Warm wash, minimum spin. Very helpful.

Why should food be any different? We don't eat socks: their effect on health is slightly more remote than food. Yet in comparison we are given more information about their composition than the food we eat, for which there is no adequate consumer protection legislation. Until food is properly labelled, how can the public make a healthy choice?

Nowhere is the need greater than with fats and oils. We eat over 4 oz of fats every day. By world standards that is a great deal. The obvious sources of fats are butter, margarine, lard, oils and visible fat on meats. Less obvious is the fat in milk, cheese, biscuits, cakes, meat products, pies, ice creams and snacks. Fat finds its way into all kinds of foods. We need to know how much fat there is, and what kind of fat it is.

The guide that follows is written to help you choose the healthiest fats, despite the inadequacy of food labels.

Fats Versus Oils

Fats and oils are both made of fatty material. The only difference is that fats are solid at room temperature, and oils are liquid. If you live in the tropics, butter becomes an oil. If you live in Greenland, olive oil becomes a fat.

Many people think that the simple difference between fats and oils is enough to tell you what to buy and eat. Word has got around that fats are bad, oils are good. In fact it is not as simple as that. As a rule fats are unhealthy, and it is also true that many oils are healthy; but some oils are not much better than fats, either because they are unhealthy in the first place, or because they have been made unhealthy by processing.

That is why it is worth knowing about the meaning of various terms much discussed by scientists and the media lately, and even sometimes to be seen on food labels: 'saturated', 'monounsaturated', 'polyunsaturated', 'fatty acids', 'hydrogenated' and 'essential fats'. And a new term, 'trans fatty acids' may be making a greater public appearance.

All fats and oils are made of fatty acids, of which there are over twenty different types. No form of edible fat or oil is made up of only one fatty acid. It is the relative proportion of the different fatty acids in a fat or oil that makes it solid or liquid; healthy, unhealthy, or neutral; easily stored or liable to go rancid; smelly or odourless.

There are three classes of fats, or fatty acids: these are, saturated, monounsaturated, and polyunsaturated. Saturated fats are sometimes called SFAs (saturated fatty acids) and polyunsaturated fats are sometimes called PUFAs (polyunsaturated fatty acids).

All fatty acids have a complex chemical structure: they are made up of chains of carbon atoms, to which hydrogen and oxygen atoms are bound. When the chemical structure is relatively simple, and when the carbon atoms have a high proportion of hydrogen atoms bound to them, the fatty acid is saturated (that is, saturated with hydrogen). When the structure is relatively complex, more carbon atoms are free from hydrogen atoms, and so the fatty acid is unsaturated (that is, unsaturated with hydrogen). Such fatty acids also either have what is known as one 'double bond' within the chain of carbon atoms at some point (in which case they are 'monounsaturated') or more than one 'double bond', in which case they are 'polyunsaturated'. The meaning of 'saturated' or 'unsaturated' – with hydrogen – is worth remembering.

When a fat or oil is referred to as being 'saturated' or 'highly saturated' that means that it contains a high proportion of saturated fatty acids. Conversely, when a fat or oil is referred to as being 'polyunsaturated' or 'high in polyunsaturates' that means that it contains a high proportion of polyunsaturated fatty acids.

Saturated Fats

Which fats and oils are saturated? What do they do to the body? No saturated fat is essential for health. Most scientific debate about fats and health has centered on the connection between saturated fats and heart disease. There is increasing evidence that saturated fats may cause a variety of other diseases, notably breast cancer, the biggest single killer cancer among women of all ages. Saturated fats may also cause various disorders and diseases of the gut and vital organs.

These are the saturated fats to watch for:

Dairy fats	– butter, cheese, fat on top of milk, single and double cream
Meat fats	– beef, lamb, pork, bacon, suet, lard, dripping
Processed fats	– many margarines and cooking fats, some blended vegetable oils, many fats used in industry to make cakes, biscuits, pies, snacks, sausages, etc.
Plant oils	– coconut oil, palm oil

All these fats tend to be highly saturated. Saturated fats are unhealthy because they make the blood more sticky and more likely to get 'stuck' on the arterial walls. Furthermore, saturated fats damage the structure of the arterial walls, causing rigidity and lumpy obstructions. Sticky blood is more likely to clot on the lumps. Atherosclerosis, the name given to this process of deterioration, happens slowly over many years, usually decades, and we cannot feel it happening. But it can kill by causing such a big obstruction that the blood cannot get through. If the obstruction happens in one of the heart arteries, we have a heart attack.

Saturated fat causes and accelerates atherosclerosis. This is a condition which begins in childhood. By the end of our lives, 90 per cent of us suffer from atherosclerosis. Half of us will develop symptoms as a result of it: angina (pains in the chest), circulatory problems, heart attacks. A quarter of us will die from it, many before we are sixty-five. The UK has the highest rate of premature death and illness (before sixty-five years) from heart disease in the world. The saturated fat we eat is a major underlying cause.

Monounsaturated Fats

In the 'bad', 'middling' and 'good' stakes, monounsaturated fats are middling – neutral, neither good nor bad for our health, as far as anybody knows. As far as heart disease is concerned, they neither make blood more sticky nor less sticky; they neither cause nor prevent atherosclerosis.

On average we consume just about as much mono-unsaturated fats as saturated fatty acids. As far as food is concerned, fats and meats that are high in monounsaturates are bad or good for us, according to what other fats they contain. About half of beef fat or lard is monounsaturated, for example – but almost all the rest of these fats are saturated and unhealthy. On the other hand, almost half of mackerel oil or peanut oil is monounsaturated – but much of the rest is healthy polyunsaturates. The outstanding example of an oil high in monounsaturates is olive oil, the key to the health of the peoples of the Mediterranean for thousands of years. Science still has much to learn about food and health, and it may even be that olives have an 'ingredient x' in them which makes them especially good for health. Their secret almost certainly is that, while olive oil is about 70 per cent monounsaturates, it is also 10–15 per cent polyunsaturates, of which most is linoleic acid, a specific example of a polyunsaturated fat which is an 'essential fat', vital to life and health as a vitamin is (more about essential fats later).

The Greeks eat large quantities of olive oil, yet do not often develop heart disease, nor many of the disorders and diseases from which we suffer in Britain. The best olive oil is called 'extra-virgin' which comes from the first pressing of the fruit. It is rich, thick and dark green, with a delicious flavour. Olive oil can be used without harm in cooking. And it won't make you fat provided you take regular exercise.

Polyunsaturated Fats and Essential Fats

Because the polyunsaturates are the good guys, and now are increasingly often mentioned by name, it is worth mentioning the ones that are often talked about: linoleic acid, and linolenic acid. Humans cannot make these, therefore food has to supply them. In addition there are others such as eicosapentaenoic acid and arachidonic acid, which the body manufactures from linoleic and linolenic acids, and which are found in fatty fish and offals.

Polyunsaturates are good for our health. In particular, they protect against heart disease: they make the blood less sticky and less likely to clot. This is why the people in the USA have gone over to polyunsaturates in such a big way. It is possible even that polyunsaturates may in time repair some of the damage done to the walls of arteries (atherosclerosis) by saturated fats: animal experiments have produced encouraging results.

People in the West consume a lot of fats, and the NACNE target of 30 per cent of calories from fats (down from the current 40 per cent or so) still leaves us eating a lot of fat compared with other countries. In Japan, for example, the figure used to be a mere 10 per cent, and even with Westernisation is only about 20 per cent of calories from fats.

Essential fats are not only good for us, they are vital to health and life itself. For this reason essential fats are sometimes termed 'vitamin F'. One particular distinguished British scientist, Dr Hugh Sinclair, has made essential fats his life's work, and it is only very recently that his own observations have been recognized as being of crucial importance, and verified by other researchers.

It may be that many people in Britain (and other Western countries) are seriously short of essential fats. The brain and the central nervous system, including the soft part of the spinal column, are made mostly from essential fats, which therefore can be seen both as the source of, and the food for, our mental and physical intelligence.

A series of diseases of the brain and central nervous system are disturbingly common in Britain. These include mental retardation from birth and multiple sclerosis. These currently are regarded as 'mystery diseases' of unknown cause. It is too early to be sure that these diseases have lack of essential fats as a cause. But deficiency of essential fats will certainly only do harm to the brain and central nervous system; and many people in Britain are indeed short of essential fats. The problem is food processing.

Where are polyunsaturates and essential fats to be found? The foods we call 'fats' and think of as British by tradition — butter, suet, dripping, lard — do all contain small amounts of polyunsaturates, but are also very highly saturated. The following oils and fats contain large amounts of polyunsaturates or are low in saturated fats. These are the ones to buy and eat, either as the whole food (for example: fatty fish, seeds, nuts) or as the extracted oil:

corn (maize) oil
sesame oil
soya oil
sunflower oil
safflower oil
olive oil
fish oils (unprocessed, unhardened)
walnut oil
margarines labelled high 'in polyunsaturates'

Tiny amounts of essential fats are found in nearly all whole foods. In grain, the essential fats are in the germ (which is of course part of wholegrain – wholemeal – bread, but which is eliminated in the making of white flour and therefore white bread). In fruit, in almost all cases the essential fats are concentrated in the peel, pith and seeds (which we tend to discard and are eliminated in fruit juices). Nuts and seeds are rich in essential fats. Some beans, for example soya beans, are good sources of essential fats, when eaten whole. Ancient communities of hunters and gatherers, and their present day counterparts, rely on these tiny amounts of essential oils. Added together, they are an important source of healthy fats in their food. Many settled peasant communities also have very little visible fats in their food. The oils in nuts, seeds, fruit and green leaves are important for them too.

What about aninals? Like us, animals are what they eat. Sedentary people in the West who eat a lot of fats become over-fat; and their body fat itself is composed largely of saturated fats if that is what they have eaten. So is the muscle flesh of over-fat people: it becomes shot through with fatty streaks and layers also high in saturated fats. The same process happens to animals that are confined, and fed food concentrates. The bodies of unhealthy animals are largely made up of unhealthy fat (water and bones aside). In sharp contrast, animals that are fit, and eat foods high in essential fats, are first of all lean and muscular; and second, what fat they do have is itself high in essential fats.

The message, if you eat meat, is therefore to eat the meat of creatures that in life lived free. Above all, perhaps this means fish. But also game birds and animals are good choices: pigeon, grouse, pheasant, deer (venison), hare, rabbit, – the choice depends on your taste and pocket. With fish the best choice is fatty fish: the despised mackerel, sprat and herring, fresh sardines, trout, tuna and salmon. All these are high in essential oils. One in particular, eicosapentaenoic acid, has a protective effect on the circulation. This explains why traditionally some societies have eaten a lot of meat or fish and yet not had any problems with heart disease. Eskimos, for example, eat fish and seal meat as their staple food (or did, before the trading posts arrived). The traditional Eskimo diet is very high in essential fats and low in saturated fats.

The Horrors of Hydrogenation

But how can it be that we in Britain eat far more fat than our ancestors, and yet are at risk of being short of essential fats? The problem is food processing.

A great nutritionist once said, 'the only good food is food that goes bad'. To put it another way: the more life there is in a food the better it is for our health. But death follows life. Like a human body, an animal or vegetable body 'goes bad' after being slaughtered or plucked: it rots, becomes putrid, gets infested, grows mould, attracts poisons. And essential fats become rancid. Saturated fats, by contrast, are stable: they 'keep'.

Apply all this to biscuits, for example. The British are very partial to biscuits.

After his sojourn in Northern Ireland, James Prior MP did not take the Chiltern Hundreds – he took the biscuit, rejoining the Board of United Biscuits. Look at biscuits, all made with fats, from the point of view of Mr Peek, Mr Frean, Mr McVitie, and Mr Prior (or cakes, come to that, from the point of view of Mr Kipling). A biscuit needs to be reliable. That means that it needs to stay tasty and crisp, and taste the same, on Monday, Friday, and the next ten or twelve Mondays also. What that means is 'shelf-life'.

In its protective casing a nut or a seed, or a dried bean or legume, stays fresh. But as soon as the oil is extracted, it starts to oxidize in the air. It loses its stability and eventually goes rancid. But with cakes, biscuits, crisps, confectionery, cooking fats, margarines, meat products, and all such foods using fats, what is wanted is a uniform, reliable product that 'keeps'; and that usually means hydrogenation.

When the food manufacturing industry uses fats and oils to make margarines, cooking fats and oils, fats for biscuit and cake manufacture, crisps, sweets, etc., they are first processed. This is what happens. The fats and oils are extracted from the parent plant or animal material, washed, bleached, filtered, deodorized and decoloured. Furthermore they may then be hydrogenated (hardened). They can go through more than fifteen different processes, with a variety of different chemicals added to them at each step. The net effect is a product without smell or taste, cleaned and purified of toxic material, a product of uniform and quite specific viscosity and texture. These processes make it possible for your favourite margarine always to look, taste and feel the same, but you might be surprised to learn that its ingredients may change from batch to batch. The fats- and oils-processing industry usually uses whichever fats are cheapest on the world market. Then they turn them into the uniform products we have come to expect.

The food industry too expects uniformity of ingredients: biscuit-manufacturing plants wouldn't be too happy if the fats they used turned out to be a different consistency each week. Try creating the filling for a wafer biscuit with a liquid oil.

The tendency with all processing of fats and oils is to make them more saturated, by hydrogenation. Whenever you see the label 'contains hydrogenated vegetable oils', this means that liquid oils have been heated with hydrogen in order to fill the double bonds in the fatty acids. Hydrogenation makes the fat or oil more solid and more saturated. It can turn a healthy oil into a harmful product. Nearly all of the fats and oils used in food processing have been hydrogenated.

Brand loyalty is the name of the game. Business requires any branded product to seem to be exactly the same whenever purchased. (Within the industry, brilliant minds are always at work, finding ways to degrade the product and yet make it appear identical.) But, over all, fats in processed foods are hydrogenated. The food industry does not use them in order to poison the population, but for the simple and imperative reason that saturated fats 'keep' (particularly if they are helped along with a few of those E-numbered preservatives). The biscuit-buying public does not want to buy a cream cracker with niffy cream and soggy cracker. The grocer does not want mouldy biscuits with greasy labels. So, we are saturated with saturated fats.

Trans Fatty Acids

The hydrogenation of fats produces another undesirable change, which worried the Department of Health in its 1984 report on diet and cardiovascular disease. Processing changes some of the polyunsaturated fats into 'trans polyunsaturated fatty acids', which has the effect of altering their behaviour in the human body. Put simply, trans polyunsaturated fatty acids behave rather like saturated fats, even though they are still polyunsaturated in structure. The processing has the effect of making the fatty acid 'flip over' into a mirror image of itself. A healthy, naturally occurring 'cis' fatty acid flips into an unhealthy 'trans' fatty acid which interferes with the metabolism of healthy essential fats in the body. Trans fatty acids are found in margarines, blended and mixed vegetable oils, and in the hydrogenated fats used to make cakes and biscuits. Small quantities of 'trans' fats are also found in dairy fat, but it is food processing which produces the largest quantities. Some margarines contain about 6 per cent trans fats.

This is as yet one more reason to buy good quality oils, and only to use those margarines which say 'high in polyunsaturates' on the label, because they tend to contain less trans fats than the more saturated varieties.

Margarines

How do you get liquid oil to set in a tub, or stay in a paper packet? Harden it, of course. And that is just what the manufacturers do to make margarine.

The process was invented in the nineteenth century by Mege-Mouriès, a Frenchman who was asked by the Victualling Department of the French Navy to make a cheap substitute for butter. In 1869 the process was patented in Britain, and it was not long before margarine became the poor man's butter. It definitely had an inferior status.

Today things are rather different, because all the indications are that the British public, in common with many of its European neighbours, increasingly believes that margarine is a more healthy product than butter. Starting in 1981, we bought more margarine than butter for the first time since the Second World War.

Today the majority of margarines are made with a variety of different fats and oils – fish oils, soya oil, sunflower oil, corn oil, palm oil, coconut oil, lard. In fact, anything cheap is used. But the better quality margarines are increasingly being made of one type of oil alone. Most margarines are now made with vegetable fats only, so you might be tempted to think that they contain few harmful saturated fats. But beware of labels which tell you that a margarine is made of '100 per cent vegetable oil'. This does not necessarily mean that it is healthy: it could still be highly saturated.

When margarines are made, the raw fats and oils go through all the processes already listed. Deodorization is very important if fish oil is included. Then the fats are mixed with water, together with emulsifying agents to stop the mixture separating. Margarines in Britain must by law contain added vitamins A and D. The 'vitaminized' mixture is coloured, flavoured, salted and then poured into tubs or set in blocks. The final mixture must by law have a fat content of not less than 80 per cent, and a water content of not more than 16 per cent. It usually contains 2 per cent salt.

How can you know what margarine contains? We are back to the old sock problem, because, unlike socks, the manufacturers are not required to tell us which fats they have used to make the stuff nor the quantities of different fats used, nor the degree of saturation. The result is that amidst the margarine jungle many of us are hopelessly confused. Nearly all of us are ignorant, through no fault of our own.

Which margarines should you choose? Only buy ones labelled 'high in polyunsaturates'. That way you know they are more likely to be low in harmful saturates.

New food labelling regulations were laid before Parliament on 29 August 1984. They came into effect on 19 September 1984, with enforcement from 1 January 1986. They say that any food which claims to be 'high in polyunsaturates' must fulfil the following conditions:

   i. The food must contain at least 35 per cent fat by weight (in other words a manufacturer cannot say a comparatively low-fat food is high in polyunsaturates)

  ii. At least 45 per cent of the fat must be polyunsaturates

 iii. Not more than 25 per cent of the fat must be saturates

 iv. Any claim that the food is high in polyunsaturates must be accompanied by the words 'low in saturates' or 'low in saturated fatty acids'

  v. The food must be labelled with the total quantity of fat present, the amount of polyunsaturated fats and the amount of saturated fats, expressed as a percentage weight of the food.

Avoid all margarines not labelled in this way. Many people have also been confused by claims about cholesterol content. A margarine that is low in cholesterol is not necessarily any better than its next door neighbour on the shelf. Most margarines are made from hardened vegetable oils which contain no cholesterol in the first place. However, they may be heavily saturated.

The 1984 labelling regulations say that any claims about the cholesterol content of a food must comply with the following rules:

i. The cholesterol content must be not more than 0·0005 per cent of cholesterol (by weight)

ii. The manufacturer must also make a claim about polyunsaturates (in other words the fatty acid composition must comply with all the rules set out, as above)

iii. Any claim about the absence of cholesterol, or its low level, must not be accompanied by any suggestion that the food is beneficial to human health.

So until January 1986, all manufacturers are bringing their labelling into line with these rules. And the consumer will at least have information with which to make an informed choice.

As for the actual ingredients of margarine, some manufacturers have developed a clever technique to make you think that their product is better than it really is. 'Made with 100 per cent sunflower oil' it says on top of the tub. Turn it round and look at the list of contents: 'sunflower oil, hydrogenated plant or vegetable oils . . . etc'. So although what sunflower oil there is is indeed 100 per cent sunflower and nothing else, there are other oils as well! This sort of attractive label is supposed to make you think the product is healthier than others – which it may be or may not be. Remember, the quality of a margarine depends on the starting material and the degree of hydrogenation.

Butter Versus Margarine – Which Should You Use?

The margarine and butter advertising people have fought it out in newspapers and magazines and on TV about the 'naturalness' of butter and the alien modern processes by which margarine is made (those are the arguments of the Butter Information Council); and the implied health benefits of polyunsaturates and the purity of the oils used (that's the margarine people). However, when it comes to misusing scientific information, neither side has a clean track record. They are in it for the money. The butter people are desperately trying to encourage us to eat our way through the million-tonne EEC butter mountain, made ever bigger by falling sales as customers switch to margarines for economic as well as health reasons; while the margarine people are doing their best to expand their share of the market.

What should you do? First, if the choice is between conventional British margarines and butter, forget it. Most of these 'old-fashioned' margarines and some of the newer ones are highly saturated. Krona, for example, is one of the most saturated margarines on the market. However, many of the newer margarines, soft and labelled 'high in polyunsaturates' (not just Flora, but many 'own brands' as well), are much lower in saturated fats than butter. If you intend to continue spreading your bread and potatoes thickly with either, then a good polyunsaturated margarine is preferable.

But do you really need to eat a lot of butter or margarine in the first place? The French, Italians, Greeks, Portuguese and Indians wouldn't dream of smothering their bread with a layer of fat. Bread just isn't eaten like that. So why do we do it? Partly it must have something to do with our eating habits in the nineteenth century. Bread and dripping was all many people had, and the habit has stuck. The other problem is the quality of our bread, of which more later. If as a nation we had access to good-quality bread which merited pride of place on the dining table, would we need to hide it underneath a layer of fat? The fact is that most British bread just isn't fit to eat on its own. Would you have the nerve to present an Italian or a Greek with a plateful of white sliced Sunblest or Mothers Pride?

Buy good bread and you will be halfway towards discovering how to eat less fat. Never mind the extra cost: it balances out as you spend less on the butter and margarine, less on meats and less on highly processed foods.

Another area of confusion about butter, margarines, fats and oils is their calorie or energy value. Many people believe that margarine is 'more slimming' than butter. In fact butter has 740 calories per 100 grams, and margarines have 730 calories per 100 grams. Oils have more, 899 calories per 100 grams, but only because they contain less water.

Low-Fat Spreads

Fats labelled 'low-fat spreads' contain fewer calories. Examples are Gold or Outline, which have less than half the energy value of butter or margarine. The manufacturers are not permitted to call them 'butter' or 'margarine' which by law have to have a higher fat content. These products only contain about half the fat of butter or margarine, plus some water and something like gelatine to stick it all together so that it looks like margarine rather than an unappetising oil slick. St. Ivel's Gold is one of the highest in polyunsaturated fatty acids.

Cholesterol In Food

Cholesterol is the substance that builds up in the arteries and causes blockages in the circulation. It is manufactured in our livers, and also comes from our food. Chemically it is rather like a fat.

Too much saturated fat in food results in extra cholesterol being made in the liver, and this leads to too much cholesterol circulating in the blood. The cholesterol is then deposited in the arterial walls. In addition, cholesterol derived from food can be deposited in the arterial walls, and it has been shown that cholesterol-rich diets do raise the blood cholesterol level in some people.

Reducing the level of blood cholesterol brings about a decrease in the rate of death from heart attacks. This has been demonstrated in large population studies.

Cholesterol is only found in animal foods. Plants contain none. The foods that supply most cholesterol are egg yolks and offal (brains are particularly high in cholesterol). It is found in meat, and red meat contains more than poultry; and also in cream, cream on top of milk, lard, suet, butter, cheese, sausages and other meat products. Generally speaking, the more animal fat a food contains, the higher the level of cholesterol.

Reducing saturated fats in our food will have the effect of reducing cholesterol as well, because the two things are so often found together.

But how many eggs should you eat? Egg yolks contain cholesterol, fat, protein, minerals and vitamin A. The whites contain no fats, no cholesterol, some proteins and minerals. It is the egg yolks that are the problem as far as cholesterol is concerned. It is best to eat an average of no more than three or four eggs a week, and that includes the eggs used in baking and in manufactured foods (cakes, biscuits, sauces).

Butter, Margarines, Fats and Oils – A Summary of the Advice

- Fry less. Grill more.

- Use less fats in cooking.

- Use less lard and dripping.

- Buy only margarines and cooking fats labelled 'high in poly-unsaturates'.

- Use these oils: sunflower, safflower, corn (maize), soya, olive, walnut, sesame.

- Avoid 'blended' or 'mixed' vegetable oils.

- Spread butter/margarine thinner on bread.

- Eat no more than three to four eggs a week.

- Buy better quality bread. Wholemeal is best.

- Stop putting butter on vegetables.

CHAPTER 2

Meat and Poultry

OUR ANCESTORS: HUNTERS OR GATHERERS?
FATTY MEAT – BY ORDER. SAUSAGES: THE BANGER EXPLODED.
WHAT MEAT IS BEST TO EAT?

We have been brought up to think of meat as a positive benefit to health. Bulging with protein, meat goes at the top of most health visitors' lists of good food for growing children. The more meat the better. Man is a carnivore and cannot live without it. That's what we have been taught.

An analysis of the average British diet gives a very different picture. We eat too much fat in this country, and nearly one third of that surplus fat comes from meat. Furthermore, not only is our meat fatty, but between two fifths and a half of red meat fat is saturated – in other words, very unhealthy. The benefit that meat provides is very often outweighed by its high saturated fats content.

The most saturated meat fat comes from beef and lamb, followed by pork, then poultry. The general advice in this book is to reduce your consumption of meat fat by eating smaller quantities of leaner cuts. This need not cost more, because you can compensate by buying less.

In Britain, as in most other countries, meat dishes have a mark of prestige. The more meat you can afford, the more contented your guests, the higher your social standing. This is what we have been taught. However, our attitude is changing. For as vegetarianism and 'ethnic' cooking take over in middle-class neighbourhoods, word is getting round not only that large quantities of meat are not essential, but also that we might even be healthier without it.

This book is not concerned with promoting a vegetarian way of life. It is concerned with good health, and the two are not of necessity linked. For over four million years, humankind has lived on and adapted to an astonishingly varied diet: fruits, nuts, seeds, berries, leaves, roots, molluscs, crustaceans, insects, fish and mammals of all sizes. The number of plants and animals that we regard today as 'food' is small by comparison with eating habits in traditional 'hunting and gathering' societies.

Our Ancestors: Hunters or Gatherers?

Our ancestors probably ate far more plant foods and far less meat than the ancient men so beloved of children's ency-clopedias: hairy, roaring creatures brandishing their clubs and canines, tearing through the pages in pursuit of man-sized game. The truth was in all probability somewhat less spec-tacular. Studies of hunting and gathering communities alive today, and of fossil remains of the ancient settlements, indicate that the emphasis was on the gathering rather than the hunting. Much of our ancestors' food was vegetable; meats were chiefly from small creatures – insects, crustaceans (like shellfish, crabs), molluscs (like snails), worms and rodents. Catching a wild bison would be a bit of a problem without good weapons. Even with the development of effective weapons and traps, considerable patience and plenty of luck are needed to get a good catch of monkey or wild goat.

Most ancient communities relied heavily on plant foods, although it is difficult to generalize, because some groups, such as the Eskimo, were quite clearly more reliant on animals than others. The Eskimo traditionally ate a lot of fish and seal meat, but supplemented it with berries, plants, roots and seaweeds.

In 1984 it was announced that a large group of Aborigines had been discovered in Australia. They had had no previous contact with white civilization, and were reported to be 'living healthily on kangaroo, snails and other animals'. Studies of Australian Aborigines show an enormous range of foods are eaten, the women providing the largest part of the food by gathering plants and lizards, insects, shellfish, crabs and small fish. Men hunt kangaroos, emus, wombats, large fish and other animals.

Peasant agriculturists rely on plant foods, but again there are exceptions, of which the Masai of East Africa are the most widely quoted. It is not commonly realized that cattle were introduced to Africa only 4,000 years ago, probably via Egypt and Ethiopia. The Masai, Samburu and Karamajong have based a culture on their cattle which not only supply food, but also are a sign of wealth. These people drink milk, mixed with blood, and cultivate grain crops. They also gather seeds, fruits and leaves from their surroundings.

Today there are few ancient communities which remain uncontaminated by modern habits. Collecting together all that we now know about ancient humankind, it is clear that the quality of their food was very different from our own. Large-scale intensive cultivation of plants, genetic manipulation, the fattening of largely sedentary animals, the preservation of food with salt and in cans – all these things have helped to increase the number of people wandering about on the earth. But what of their biological quality? Here again, a look at meats eaten by ancient peoples is instructive, for it could show us how to improve our food in the future.

Fat Pigs for Fat Pigs

Consider for a moment the average factory-fed twentieth-century pig: suckled briefly at birth, then removed for intensive feeding at a rate calculated for maximum deposition of edible tissue, with no seasonal variations in food supply and no space to run around. What sort of animal does this produce? A creature as unfit as the humans who consume it, this pig would get out of breath running across a field. Yet the wild boar spends its day exercising, in pursuit of food and escaping danger. Man and pig, we are all in the same predicament: twentieth-century inertia.

Present-day intensive feeding methods, the sorts of food animals are fed, and their lack of exercise, all help to produce fatty animals far removed from the condition of their wild ancestors. Meat produced by twentieth-century methods is not only fatter than wild game; the fat is also higher in harmful saturated fats and lower in polyunsaturated fats.

Genetic breeding and manipulation of animal feeds have done a lot in recent years to reduce the fat of carcasses, particularly pigs, but we have a long way to go. It is doubtful whether improved genetics and healthier feeding will ever be able to reproduce the quality of meat caught in the wild.

Fatty Meat – By Order

One reason why our meat is so fatty is that government regulations actually encourage its production. The Ministry of Agriculture's carcass grading standards specify the minimum quantity of fat on an animal. Unless the carcass comes up to the minimum, it is rejected as unfit for human consumption. These minimum standards encourage farmers to fatten their animals in order to get a better price at slaughter. Through EEC and government subsidies and in our weekly food purchased, we foot the bill for this wasteful and harmful practice. Fat costs money to produce. If the Ministry of Agriculture took the nation's health into consideration when deciding on policy, we would all be in better shape.

The Department of Health COMA report, *Diet and Cardio-*

vascular Disease (July 1984), advised the government that 'consideration should be given to ways and means of encouraging the production of leaner carcasses in sheep, cattle and pigs (for example by adjustments to the operation of the carcass grading systems).' The Minister of Agriculture made a small move in this direction in March 1985. And there are signs that the Meat and Livestock Commission is thinking about this problem, and considering how leaner meat could be produced.

So what sort of meat do we eat, and in what quantities?

As incomes rose after the Second World War, the nation as a whole took to the joint of meat. The population increased, the farmers flourished. Meat consumption went up by 16 per cent between 1955 and 1980. Lamb and beef actually declined by 32 per cent and 14 per cent respectively, while pork went up by 77 per cent. And then there is the meteoric rise of the battery chicken – an increase in consumption of 1,229 per cent in thirty years! We now consume about 5½ oz of meat (raw weight) each day: about 1 oz of beef, 1 oz of poultry, ½ oz each of pork, lamb and bacon and nearly 2 oz of meat products – pies, sausages, processed meats.

How much fat is in the meat you buy? Unless you always buy lean meat, the answer is quite a lot. And even 'lean' meat does contain fats, because today's agricultural production methods ensure that muscle flesh becomes streaked with fatty deposits, invisible to the naked eye. So eating unlimited quantities of steak is not a good idea. If you cut the visible fat off fatty meat, you dispose of perhaps half of the fats. Poultry and game contain by far the least fat. By comparison, lean beef is rather fatty. Sausages and pies come in for a grilling later.

MEAT: THE BIG TREAT?

In general, to reduce saturated fats, aim to eat smaller quantities of lean meat. It does cost more per pound, but you do not need a lot, and there are plenty of ways to cook large dishes with little meat. Regard meat as a flavouring for the vegetables, rather than as the main item on the plate. Use smaller quantities of lean meat in stews and casseroles. Cut off all visible fat. Spread the meat out with potatoes, aubergines, carrots, peppers, pasta, rice etc., and skim the fat off the top when it is cooked. In fact eat the kind of food we all know is healthy – good old-fashioned stews and 'peasant' dishes.

Does this kind of meal take longer to cook than the traditional Sunday roast? No – but the work order is reversed. Cooking the Sunday joint is easy until you get to the end when you have to spend ten to fifteen minutes making the gravy and Yorkshire pudding and cooking the cabbage. Until then, all you do is switch on the oven, sit down and read the papers. Cooking a stew means you spend the ten to fifteen minutes at the beginning chopping up the vegetables. You still get to read the papers while it is cooking. It is not the case that healthy meat dishes necessarily take longer to prepare.

Beef, Lamb, Pork

With 'carcass' meats – beef, lamb, pork – the idea is to eat less fat. Say a total of 10 oz of lean meat per person per week rather than the present 15 oz. But it must be *lean*.

Butchers could help us to eat less meat fats by carving their carcasses in a different way. Traditional British butchering requires that the meat is cut across the muscle blocks, leaving layers of fat in between. When the muscles are rolled into joints, the fat gets rolled up with them. Continental butchery, on the other hand, dissects the muscles from the fat, and when you ask for meat, lean meat is what you get.

The new 1984 Meat Products and Spreadable Fish Products Regulations include a regulation of which all shoppers should now be aware. It says that all raw meat must be labelled with a declaration of any added water, in the following way: 'with not more than x% added water'.

The Food Standards Committee of the Ministry of Agriculture reviewed the use of added water in carcass meat in its 1980 report. It said, 'The use of techniques . . . make it possible for the meat processor to add water together with other substances to meat without any obvious visible changes occurring. This applies equally to fresh or to cured meats.' And 'The use of materials to increase the water content of meat in such a way that the treated whole meat cuts are difficult to distinguish visually from untreated meat, is in our view to be condemned as serving no useful purpose, being intrinsically deceptive and offering an unwarranted competitive advantage.' It then discussed how such practices could be banned, but decided against such a recommendation for several reasons:

i.   Meat with anything added to it becomes a 'meat product', by definition (MAFF definition). And meat products are permitted to have added water
ii. Tenderizing agents and some additional water could make cheap, tough meat more acceptable
iii. The curing of ham and pork shoulder with salts and water is now a traditional process
iv. Poultry flesh 'sucks up' water when it is washed, so the imposition of a ban on added water in carcass meat while permitting the wetting of poultry would be inconsistent.

The Food Standards Committee therefore decided to recommend that instead of banning the practice of pumping water into meat joints, such products should be labelled when water had been added to them; the recommendation is now law.

This is how food is, legally, debased. Why has the Ministry of Agriculture allowed meat to be 'diluted' in this way? A manufacturer can now pump a joint with water, and sell it as such, provided it is labelled with the added water content.

How is the consumer to know which joint of meat is best value for money? Which among us can do the mental arithmetic, standing in a shop, to compare a beef joint with 6 per cent added water at £x per pound, with a beef joint with no added water at £y per pound? Are manufacturers now to be allowed to dilute milk provided they write it on the label? Or butter? Or oranges? For there are plenty of arguments that can be dreamed up to justify doing this sort of thing.

What seems to happen in the meat industry (and indeed in most branches of food technology) is that new processes are invented which have the effect of spinning out expensive meat into a larger volume. When the practice becomes sufficiently widespread, the Ministry of Agriculture enshrines it in legislation. This is called technological progress, which MAFF is anxious not to impede. But surely not just any old progress will do? If the meat industry were really working with their customers' interests at heart, such practices as adding water to fresh meat would not happen.

Debasement of meat quality is part and parcel of the debasement of cooking which is encouraged by many of today's convenience foods. 'Meat' is a lump of meat on a plate, the more of it the better. The trouble is that not many parts of the carcass lend themselves to such simple cookery, which is where the polyphosphates come in as tenderizing agents. As any cook knows, much meat needs to be treated and cooked with imagination, which is why poor people all round the world have traditionally discovered ways to make small amounts of the tougher cuts go further in pies and stews. With all that food science has to offer, can the manufacturers not do better than dilute our meat with water, aided and abetted with polyphosphates? And does the Ministry of Agriculture really think that this practice is in the consumer's best interest?

Chicken, Turkey and Game

Poultry and game contain less fats than carcass meats. Most of the fat is under the skin, which can be removed without spoiling the flavour when you make stews. Chicken and turkey are relatively cheap, so are a good replacement for fatty red meats and meat products.

However, be particular when you buy a chicken. For chickens are not what they used to be. Over the years they have expanded in volume and weight, and in large part it is a result of – you've guessed it – water.

The modern chicken has a complicated funeral. After being uncrated and hung on a line, it is stunned, its jugular vein is cut and it is bled. Then it is scalded before its feathers are pulled off. This is the first point where the carcass can take up water. The automatic process which takes a live chicken in at one end and puts it out at the other, frozen in a plastic bag with its giblets tucked inside, includes several washing and soaking phases. Because the bird has been drawn and plucked, water is naturally drawn into the skin.

One process in particular is giving cause for concern. The polyphosphate chicken became commonplace in the 1970s. Polyphosphates increase the amount of water taken up by the flesh. According to many of those who use them, they make the meat more tender and stop it drying out in cooking, and it carves better. This is what we are told. But the benefit to the wholesaler is really what counts, for the bird becomes heavier, and water costs a good deal less than meat! Some of the largest producers have announced that they no longer use polyphosphates in chickens. The rule is that, if used, it must be declared on the label, and if the total amount of water comes to more than 5 per cent of the finished product, that too must be declared. So if you are buying a chicken, read the ingredient list and look for polyphosphates (E450).

Under EEC regulations, water added to chickens to which no polyphosphates have been added need not be declared, even though it is well known that the water content of frozen and deep frozen chickens amounts to some 6–8 per cent of final weight. If you want a dry chicken, look for the scrawny birds.

There is one further problem caused by intensive rearing and slaughtering systems for chickens – Salmonella poisoning.

Salmonella infections are probably the most common forms of food poisoning in Britain, and chickens are one of the chief culprits. For Salmonella contamination is endemic in most modern poultry farms. Chickens pass it from one to another. At slaughter and during washing, flesh can become contaminated with water containing the bacteria, the source of which is the intestinal cavity of the bird. Each time the birds are immersed in water, during washing and soaking prior to chilling or freezing, Salmonella has a chance of being drawn into the flesh of the bird. Wet chilling is now gradually being replaced by dry chilling, which will produce a dryer bird, as well as removing one of the potential hazards of processing.

Always cook chickens, and turkeys, thoroughly. If you have cooked it once, and warm it up again, make quite sure it is well heated. And never put raw chicken next to anything which is ready to eat.

For the occasional treat, wild game is delicious, a nutritional as well as a gastronomic bonus. It is low in fats and full of flavour. Duck and goose are exceptionally fatty but they are higher in polyunsaturated fats than beef, lamb and pork.

Offal

Before considering the doubtful delights of the modern sausage and other meat products, there is one other type of meat which should briefly be mentioned. The Cinderella of the butcher's stock, offal is generally a good source of vitamins, minerals and protein and is generally low in fat. What fat it does contain is higher in essential polyunsaturates than other parts of the animal. Offal is cheap.

SAUSAGES: THE BANGER EXPLODED

The Bacon and Meat Manufacturers Association say that we each eat an average of 125 sausages every year. Given that there are 3,000 miles of coast road round Britain, one year's supply of sausages for the UK adds up to a rampart of sausages a foot wide and a foot thick, all the way round the country!

We are obviously very fond of sausages. So it might be instructive to take a look at what goes into them. Did you ever wonder as a child: just how do they make a sausage?

What is in a sausage? Does the label tell you? Next time you visit a supermarket, examine the labels of all the sausage packets you can find. Then go and take a look at the labels on tins of cat and dog food. What is the difference?

First, the cat and dog food. The manufacturers voluntarily tell you rather a lot of detail on the label about the minerals and vitamins, meat, fats, meat unfit for human consumption, ground bone, ash. Some of them give you exact amounts. Plenty of nutritional detail, so you know your Tibbles is getting his daily nourishment.

How does this compare with the sausage label? No mention of ash, bone vitamins or minerals here. No mention of fats. Just meat, pork or beef, maybe turkey (turkey? It's cheaper), possibly some vegetable fats, rusk, water, antioxidants, sodium polyphosphate, colour, flavour, flavour enhancers, monosodium glutamate, preservatives, lots of E numbers. Isn't it rather odd that manufacturers go to such lengths to tell us specifically about the nutritional value of pet food, but not that of humans?

The Dustbin of the Meat Industry

Sausages, you might be surprised to hear, often contain bone, just like dog food. The bone sausage is a relatively new invention, brought about by the development of machinery for stripping flesh off bones. Mechanically Recovered Meat (MRM to those in the business) is the name of the game. Several types of machine are in operation. Some actually crush the bone to pulp and aim to remove the soft parts by sieving. Others scrape the bones against a revolving drum, while a third type uses pressure to separate the flesh from the bone. Whichever type is used, the actual meat is effectively reduced to a pulp or 'highly pigmented slurry' as the Ministry of Agriculture described it, along with varying amounts of bone.

Apart from bone, what else finds its way into the 'traditional' sausage? First, there is fat, plenty of it. Then there may be such delectables as ground-up hides, intestines, offal, poor quality carcass meats, again carefully minced and textured so as to disguise their true origin. Does the label tell you? No, it doesn't. It simply says 'meat', and what is that supposed to mean?

Under the 1984 Meat Products and Spreadable Fish Products Regulations, the required minimum meat content for a sausage, link, chipolata or sausage meat is as follows:

i. If the name 'sausage', 'link', 'chipolata' or sausage meat' is qualified by the name 'pork' but not by the name of any other type of meat, the food must have a meat content of not less than 65 per cent of the food and a lean meat content of at least 50 per cent of the meat content of the food.

ii. In all other cases the food must have a meat content of not less than 50 per cent of the food and a lean meat content of at least 50 per cent of the meat content of the food.

In other words, a pork sausage, link, chipolata, or sausage meat, must be 65 per cent meat, and half of the meat must be lean. A beef sausage, link etc. need only be 50 per cent meat, and half of the meat must be lean.

To understand exactly what this means, we have to turn next to the regulation covering the meaning of the word 'meat'. It says:

'meat' means the flesh, including fat, and the skin, rind, gristle and sinew *in amounts naturally associated with the flesh used*, of any animal or bird which is normally used for human consumption, and includes any parts of the carcass specified in Part I of Schedule 2 which is obtained from such an animal or bird, but does not include any other part of the carcass. [Our italics].

And Part I, Schedule 2 says the following are 'meat':

> 'diaphragm, head meat (muscle meat and associated fatty tissue only), heart, kidney, liver, pancreas, tail meat, thymus, tongue'. The following are *not* to be used in uncooked meat products: 'brains, feet, large and small intestines, lungs, oesophagus, rectum, spinal cord, spleen, stomach, testicles, udder.'

In other words, putting the regulations together, a pork sausage must contain 65 per cent meat; and skin, rind, gristle and sinew, if present in that 65 per cent of meat, must only be present in proportions found in a whole pig carcass. So a sausage cannot be made of 65 per cent ground gristle, or pigs' trotters – that would be against the law. Likewise that 65 per cent of meat must not be entirely fat – also against the law, because half of the 65 per cent meat must be lean. Put into plain numbers, 32·5 per cent (one third) of the weight of a pork sausage *must* be lean meat; the next 32·5 per cent could also be lean meat, but it could equally well be fat, or a delectable mixture of gristle, sinew, diaphragm, rind and pancreas. And there is a further catch. When Public Analysts (they are in charge of checking the quality of our food) do the chemical analysis for lean meat, they assume that the 32·5 per cent lean may actually have a *further* 10 per cent fat 'naturally associated' with the lean meat! So the regulations in reality mean that a pork sausage can get away with being only 29 per cent lean meat, and a beef sausage only 22·5 per cent lean meat.

We've not finished yet! When the analyst analyses the amount of meat, one method used is to look at the amount of nitrogen in the sausage, which in turn is used to indicate the amount of protein, or lean meat present. Now it is not only muscle that contains nitrogen. So do skin and hoof and cartilage and various other bits of the body. So do some other non-meat things which sometimes find their way into a sausage. But all that matters from the manufacturers' point of view is that the sausage fits the bill as far as nitrogen is concerned. That goes down in the analysts' book as lean meat and, if the number is right, the sausage is a sausage. No matter if the lean meat is in rather short supply and the nitrogen comes from elsewhere. It passes the test.

So what is in a sausage? Who knows? The manufacturers know, but do we? The label certainly doesn't help much. No mention of the percentage of fat, hide, or skin, or bone. No mention of lean meat. Just 'meat'.

Minimum Meat

The 1984 regulations, which came into force on 12 November 1984, say that a manufacturer must declare on the label the minimum meat content. They also say that any additional fat must be listed in the ingredients. So, for example, a pork sausage which has added poultry fat or added meat fat other than pork, must have that fat declared in the list of ingredients. And the label must also tell you the other ingredients, such as rusk, water, colours, flavours, preservatives, emulsifiers. But more important to you, the consumer, is what the label does *not* tell you.

First, the meat content. How useful will it be for us to know the minimum meat content? Well, according to the Public Analysts and Trading Standards Officers, not very. There are so many ways of disguising the 'non-meat' bits as 'meat' that, for the purpose of the analysts' tests, the manufacturers have a good deal of scope for imaginative cookery. More to the point might have been a declaration of minimum *lean* meat, which according to the regulations means 'the total weight of lean meat free when raw of visible fat'. This in fact was what the Food Standards Committee recommended. From the point of view of enforcement, checking the lean meat content would be a similar problem – it still depends on the nitrogen value of the sausage. However, what the analyst *can* do is to check the fat content. This is comparatively simple. And from our point of view, a regulation governing the maximum fat content would make a lot of sense. After all, sausages are just about the most fatty kind of meat you can buy and, as such, contribute handsomely to the nation's atherosclerosis. Why did the Ministry of Agriculture then choose to ignore one of the recommendations of the Food Standards Committee whose 1980 report provided the basis for the 1984 regulations?

Their proposed definition of meat went as follows:

> meat means the flesh, and the fat, skin, rind, gristle and sinew in amounts naturally associated with the flesh used . . .

Compare this with the definition enshrined in the 1984 regulations (this almost qualifies for a 'spot the difference' competition):

> meat means the flesh, including fat, and the skin, rind, gristle and sinew in amounts naturally associated with the flesh used . . .

So the Committee recommended that fat should only be used in *amounts normally present* in a carcass. In other words, if a dressed pig carcass has 30 per cent fat, then not more than 30 per cent of the meat put into the sausage could be fat. Whereas the 1984 regulations say that 'meat' means 'flesh, *including* fat'. The phrase about the relationship to the whole carcass relates only to the skin, rind, sinew and gristle. Therefore, *meat* means *fat*! So, while a pork sausage has to have 65 per cent meat, and half (50 per cent) of it must be lean, the rest is just 'meat', and can therefore be all fat. So a pork sausage can consist of 29 per cent lean pork meat (remember the Public Analysts' 10 per cent fat), 36 per cent pork fat (equals meat, to the Ministry of Agriculture), extra poultry or other meat fat, rusk and water, together with a dose of chemical cocktail to add some nice lurid colour, sausage flavour and extra shelf life.

The point about all this is that as a nation we have a certain idea about the meaning of 'meat'. Part of our cultural heritage dictates that on the whole certain bits of the animal are not meat, that is, not eatable. Eyeballs, feet, head meat, hide, sinews, snout, lips, ears, bone – these are not usually thought of as edible meat. In other cultures they may be. It is only fair that we, the consumers, should know which bits of the body other than muscle flesh and edible offal have gone into a meat product. If the sausage industry wishes to produce bone crunch, let them promote it as such, and see if it sells. It could of course be argued that, considering the expense of meat production, as much of the carcass as possible should be used and eaten. Fair enough, but let us know what meat products contain so we can make the choice.

The 1984 regulations are, by contrast with the 1967 ones, quite specific about the other bits of a carcass that are 'meat'. But, interestingly, bone does not come into the 'non-meat' list. Nor is it listed in the 'meat' list. This means that if manufacturers are adept at grinding up bones into powder, they can put them into their sausage provided it is declared in the list of ingredients. But, in practice, what manufacturer is ever going to admit to putting ground up bones into sausages? The Trading Standards Officers and Public Analysts know this practice goes on. Their problem is to establish beyond doubt that it does happen, and to find a suitable reliable analytical test to detect the presence of bone in meat. They can test for the amount of calcium in meat products, and also for the amount of 'connective tissue' (the stringy bits that hold meat on to the bone, and the skin on to the meat) and both these measurements give a rough idea of the amount of added bone. Testing for the *exact* amount of added bone, however, is difficult, and expensive.

So 'meat', meaning muscle flesh, can be distinguished from both fat and gristle, and also to some extent from bone, but by no means do our law enforcers have an easy task. It has been extremely difficult for the Trading Standards Officers and Public Analysts to keep up with the activities of some of today's sausage makers. It remains to be seen whether the 1984 regulations will have much effect on the contents of the banger.

So far manufacturers have turned the lack of instruction in the 1967 regulations to their advantage. If it's cheap, in it goes, together with a dose of colouring, flavouring, preservative and water-holding agents, plenty of fat, plus some carefully formulated cereal rusk designed specifically to soak up the fat when you cook it, so the sausage still looks like a sausage when it's ready to eat and doesn't fall apart in the pan. It could theoretically end up being more than half fat, and still within the law. And don't forget good old plain water – nice and cheap, and heavy with it!

The Sausage of the Future

All the indications are that the post-1984 regulations sausage will be little different from the pre-1984 variety. In practice, sausages contain some one fifth to two fifths fats, the average being around a quarter (26 per cent). They usually contain about a tenth as rusk, about a half is water and the rest is 'lean' meat. But the variability is large, and you can be fairly sure that the cheaper the sausage, the more fats and water it contains. Sausages are the dustbin of the meat industry. Carcass fat and other waste products of the meat wholesale trade are always cheap, so cheap that it pays to invest in the complicated machinery needed to make today's sausage.

The Bacon and Meat Manufacturers Association (BMMA) is anxious to defend the modern sausage recipe. On the day of publication of the 1984 Department of Health's COMA Committee report, *Diet and Cardiovascular Disease*, the BMMA sent a strictly confidential letter to its members. This letter outlined the principal COMA recommendations to reduce total and saturated fats in the British diet. (It is interesting that they had copies of the report in advance. Consumer groups, doctors and MPs were denied this privilege by the DHSS.) The BMMA then offered suggestions about handling press enquiries. For example:

> Avoid accepting the report root and branch. Total acceptance would lead to difficulties . . . on how to implement the report.

And

> Fat is needed in a balanced diet. Fat makes meat tender, juicy and
> flavoursome. The meat industry believes in a balanced diet.

And here are the BMMA's suggested replies to tiresome
questions from the press, such as:

> Q: Sausages and pies contain much hidden fat. Therefore aren't
> they bad for you?
> A: They contain no more than the law permits. And sausages only
> contribute 4 per cent of total fat intake although 125 are eaten on
> average by each person in a year.

> Q: Can you buy low fat sausages and pies?
> A: Most people prefer the formulation which has been traditional
> for centuries but if there is a demand it will be met.

So there you are. Today's sausage is not more nor less than
the sausage which has been traditional for centuries! Our
historical research has obviously overlooked crucial references
to the use of polyphosphates, MRM, soya rusk, added water
and fat in 18th and 19th century documents.

Since this book was first published, some of the sausage
manufacturers have decided that the time has come for a little
improvement. In the early hours of 17 July 1984, Jonathan
Aitken MP (Conservative, Thanet South) spoke to a thinly
populated House of Commons about the need for government
action to reduce the rate of heart disease in the UK. He asked
the Minister for Health, Mr John Patten, 'to reflect for a
moment on the differences in contents labelling between a pair
of socks and a packet of sausages', both of which he held up for
all to see. (This must surely be the first time that socks and
sausages have found their way into the House of Commons.)
Mr Aitken pointed out how well the socks were labelled, in
comparison with the sausages whose label 'might be described
as a highly edited version of the contents.'

There is a long list of such contents as colour, spices, salt, and so on, but there is no mention of the quantities involved. Rather puzzlingly, there is also no mention of fat, though even an O-level chemist such as myself could easily discern a large quantity of killer fat in these sausages.

After that speech copies of Hansard veritably flew around the sausage people, and within four months, leaner sausages were on sale. Bowyer's and Wall's were first off the mark. Wall's 'Original' have no added artificial flavours. In an 'ordinary' sausage, almost three quarters of the calories come from fat, whereas in the new Wall's 'Original' just over a half of calories come from fat, a definite improvement.

It need hardly be said after all this that the majority of sausages have no place in a healthy diet. Avoid them. If you want a sausage, try the new leaner varieties, or visit your local independent butcher and continental shops and ask what goes into the mixture. If they are not prepared to tell you, buy something else instead. Look out for the minority of independent butchers and continental shops who sell sausage made with lean meat, herbs and spices, instead of fat, artificial flavouring and pink dye. Give them your support. Leaner sausages do cost more, but are healthier than their fat counterparts. Ask your supermarket manager to sell sausages which are labelled with their fat content. And don't forget to ask your children's school why they so frequently dish up such unhealthy food. Until the new 1984 Meat Product Regulations, sausages destined for catering establishments were exempt from all compositional regulations. So sausages for schools, hospitals, canteens and so on, could be made according to any old recipe the manufacturer dreamed up. Needless to say, many of them are a disgraceful product, and it will be 1986 before they have to comply with the new regulations.

MEAT PRODUCTS

A quick flip through a few of the meat industry journals is enough to convince anyone that some pretty strange things are going on in the meat products industry. The Food Standards Committee of the Ministry of Agriculture discussed these practices in some detail in its 1980 report on meat products, which formed the basis of the 1984 regulations to which all meat products (not just sausages!) have to conform. Here are just some of the common practices within today's meat industry which the committee reviewed:

> hydrated, novel protein foods
> added water/water retention
> texture changes
> tumbling and massaging
> 're-formed' meat
> Mechanically Recovered Meat
> highly pigmented slurry
> injections into meat to increase the protein content
> regenerated cellulose or plastic sausage skins.

Doesn't sound much like a traditional pork pie or meat pudding, does it? The Food Standards Committee were clearly not enamoured with many of the then (and now) current practices of the meat products industry, and they said as much in their 1980 report. Much time and money has been invested by the meat industry in developing new techniques, which, in effect, allow them to use more bits of the carcass more efficiently, and more profitably. To those destined to eat these things, the new result is meat products where the expensive 'meat' bit has been spread out as far as the manufacturers can make it go, with the addition and injection of water, rusks and vegetable proteins; chemicals to 'expand' the meat, hold the fat, maximize water addition and minimize its loss; colourings and flavourings to make you think it is meat; and preservatives to stop this mixture from breeding bacteria in a cosy watery home.

Among Trading Standards Officers there is also concern at such practices. But the Ministry of Agriculture officials clearly did not have similar feelings when they drew up the 1984 regulations, whose purpose was 'not to prohibit the use of anything', according to one civil servant.

Take one example, namely water. The addition of water to sausages, bacon, ham, and a host of other meat products (and poultry) is now very common practice. Watery meat products are the subject of frequent complaints by the public. What is the industry doing?

Quite simply, water is the cheapest thing you can put into food, apart from air. Water is not only cheap, it is also heavy, and mixed with emulsifying agents, can combine fat with other bits of the carcass to make something that looks like meat. This, of course, requires some fairly sophisticated machinery and inventive minds have been hard at work designing hardware that to you and me look more at home in a chemical factory than in a butcher's back room.

The dilution of food with water is not a new practice. Some of the earliest UK food laws were introduced to control the dilution of milk and beer, which has long been regarded as fraud. 'An Act for Preventing the Adulteration of Articles of Food or Drink' was passed in 1860, making it an offence knowingly to sell as pure or unadulterated any article of food or drink which was adulterated or not pure. The 1872 Act extended the offence to cover the mixing of food or drink with any other substance 'with intent fraudulently to increase its weight or bulk'. These early examples of legislation have been reviewed by the Ministry of Agriculture's Food Standards Committee in their 1978 report on water in food. This committee received 'strong representations' from consumer organizations about the addition of water to meat products. They said, 'We do not consider that for those foods in which the water content has deliberately been increased above the normal a mere disclosure of water in the list of ingredients would be adequate to inform and protect the consumer.'

Dilution of meat products with water is now so common that it is hard to find an undiluted ham, sausage, rasher, or slice of processed meat. The manufacturers claim that added water improves texture, which we consumers apparently like. They say that such products dry out less in cooking, apparently another benefit. They say the resulting increased tenderness and improved taste are all for our benefit. For their part, the manufacturers say it allows more efficient utilization of meat supplies, knowing full well that no one likes to see food wasted – a powerful emotive argument.

Water cannot usually be added by itself. It is necessary to use water-holding agents. Polyphosphates (E450 on the list of ingredients) give us wet meat, wet chicken, wet bacon, wet ham and wet sausages, not to mention wet fish, of which more later. If you were the Minister of Agriculture, what would you do with the polyphosphates? How many of us would not ban them? It is we the consumers who pay for this legalized debasement of food, by buying water when we really want meat. The new meat products regulations say that all water added to all raw or uncooked meat must be declared as follows: 'with not more than x% added water'. But how big will the writing be? Will you be able to do a quick calculation in the supermarket or butcher's shop, to work out the real price of watered ham with, say, 12½ per cent added water compared to its unwatered equivalent? Will you know which is better value for money? After all, it's the meat you go to buy, not the water. Who is going to safeguard fair trading for the shopper in a hurry without the ability to do this piece of arithmetic?

Waterlogged Bacon

We may soon need to wring out our bacon before we cook it! The soggy rasher is due to get even soggier. Under the new regulations, cured meats with more than 10 per cent added water must have a label 'with not more than x% added water'. Polyphosphates must also be put on the label.

Much of the bacon now sold in plastic has actually been cured in the pack. The raw meat is sliced, then packed together with a curing solution, which is why water pours out of the pack when you open it. More water spills out as the bacon warms up to room temperature, and yet more comes out on cooking, to sizzle and spit in the pan. Apparently we like our bacon wet because the texture is 'better'.

The water problem deserves to be looked at in some detail, for it demonstrates how the consumer invariably loses out on matters of food composition, when the all-important discussions are largely confined behind closed doors in Whitehall and the food factories.

The 1984 regulations say that water must be declared in uncooked cured meats if they contain more than 10 per cent water. How did the Ministry of Agriculture arrive at this figure?

The Gold Standard for bacon curing is the Wiltshire Curing Process, for which the Bacon and Meat Manufacturers have a Code of Practice. Referring to this, the Food Standards Committee Report of 1980 recommended that all uncooked cured meats should not contain more than 10 per cent curing solution without special labelling.

In the draft legislation prepared in 1981 by the Ministry of Agriculture, this was interpreted as 10 per cent *added water* before mention need be made on the label. Another 'spot the difference' competition. By 'curing solution', the Foods Standards Committee was referring not only to the water content of the solution but also the curing salts that contribute to a high proportion of its total weight. Ten per cent added water alone is the equivalent of about *15 per cent* added curing solution, leaving manufacturers the scope for pumping in about 5 per cent extra undeclared water, over and above the traditional process.

And when the BMMA's 1978 Code of Practice was revised

after the 1980 report of the Food Standards Committee, surprise, surprise, the new code allowed more water! This has since been the subject of debate among the trade and the enforcement authorities. The view of the trade is that 10 per cent added water is about right. Trading Standards Officers have said it is too much.

So now we are due to be offered even wetter bacon than before. Trading Standards Officers are not amused. But the Ministry of Agriculture have swallowed it, water and all.

Wetness apart, the modern rasher *is* less fatty than it used to be, because of changes in pig breeding. If you eat bacon often, look for lean cuts and remove the fat.

Mechanically Recovered Meat

It is not just sausages that contain MRM. The use of MRM is on the increase, despite assurances by the industry that its presence is self-limiting because of its strong colour and other undesirable qualities. This is what the Food Standards Committee said about MRM in 1980:

> MRM . . . is chemically less stable than carcass meat and presents a greater microbiological risk. It cannot simply be regarded as equivalent to carcass meat.

> The nature of the material derived . . . raises a number of questions, not least of which is the acceptability of the product to the consumer.

> We are not convinced that the material known as MRM as produced by the types of machine at present in use would be regarded by the consumer as equivalent to meat.

> MRM ranges in appearance from a highly pigmented slurry or emulsion to a coarsely ground mince-like product.

> The product may include some bone marrow and, especially if the bones have been ground before recovery, it may have a higher

calcium content than other meat, derived from fine bone particles.

MRM differs in both texture and behaviour from hand-boned meat.

And so on. The Food Standards Committee considered the problems for the consumer both as regards the nutritional quality in MRM and as regards its relationship to what we all know as meat and recommended that where MRM is used in an amount of more than 5 per cent of the declared lean meat content, there should be written on the label, 'contains x per cent Mechanically Recovered Meat'.

So what do the 1984 regulations say about MRM? Nothing. Why has the Ministry of Agriculture ignored the advice of its own Committee, whose members include independent scientists, enforcement officers and, not least, members of the food industry itself?

In the United States, where MRM is used it must be declared on the label. Moreover, its use has been prohibited in certain meat products. In the UK, MRM does not exist, at least as far as legislation is concerned.

The Government Chemist apparently has a new test for MRM which until now has been impossible to detect, except in so far as chips of bone might have been found floating about in sausages. So the days of unrestricted use of MRM may be numbered. Until then, we have no way of knowing whether we are buying meat or MRM in a meat product, so well disguised can MRM be by a meat manufacturer with a flair for design and sculpture. Its use is on the increase. Let us hope the Ministry of Agriculture will abandon its ludicrous argument that, because it cannot be detected on analysis, the use of MRM should not be limited, either by standards for food content or by better labelling.

Next on the list of undesirable practices is the inclusion of large quantities of ground pork rind in meat products. Again, the definition of meat is instructive. It only allows rind 'in amounts naturally associated with the flesh used'. In other words, the rind on a pork joint is legal. Adding pork rind to a product which has no other pork is not. Nor is the addition of large quantities of rind, plus or minus the gelatinous water in which it has been cooked.

Again, the Public Analyst is in trouble, for rind contains nitrogen, which 'analyses out' (as they put it in the trade) as 'meat'. Yet rind protein is not the same as muscle protein, and the nutritional content of its cooking water is certainly nowhere near either of them!

The most imaginative use of rind so far is dried, pulverised rind, which has a good shelf life and can be stored until required. At that point, it is rehydrated, and lo, it takes up four times its own weight of water! And the result is indistinguishable from meat flesh by the nitrogen test!

Great stuff, rind is, if you are thinking of going into the meat products industry!

Re-formed Meat

Alas, this is not what you might think. Re-formed meat is not the work of a born-again meat manufacturer. For this is where the 'tumbling and massaging' come into their own, together with a dose of polyphosphates and other agents which 'hold' water, relax the muscle fibres, and produce a gluey mess which can then be stuck together, pressed into jelly moulds, cooked, turned out, and, hey presto, a joint of ham!

Naturally, the manufacturers claim that this process is very efficient, for how else could they use up all those little flakes of wasted meat and fat? The Food Standards Committee took the view that 'the consumer should be told when re-formed or restructured meat is used'. And they weren't too happy about the use of 'protein-bearing' ingredients in such products, which 'analyse out' as nitrogen, but are not meat. In particular, vegetable proteins, such as soya, have been used in re-formed meat products, without declaration on the label. And so have cereal proteins.

The regulations say that all ingredients must be declared on the label. But without precise ingredient labelling, giving precise quantities, how are we to know what is being put into our food? Which products are better value for money? It is about time the legislation was reformed, to take account of some of the peculiar practices in today's re-formed meat manufacturing. Next time you pick up a perfectly formed steak or chop, take a closer look. It may have been born again.

Chamber of Horrors

A *wonderful* new machine has appeared on the market. It crushes up anything, absolutely anything, except teeth, put through it! This terrific invention is a godsend to the petfood manufacturers; but surely they couldn't be contemplating its use for human food? Could they? Surely not! Whole pigs' heads? Snout . . . lips . . . eyeballs . . . bones . . . ears? (And it is indistinguishable from meat when the Public Analyst does his test . . .)

And so it goes on. And on. And on. Meat is expensive. All these practices allow more extensive and more efficient use of the carcass. More often than not, such processes are pioneered by the less reputable branches of the meat trade, leading others to follow suit lest they get left behind in today's competitive market. Any large-scale manufacturer producing and selling meat products containing no added water, no polyphosphates, no bones, no added rind, no artificial colours or flavours, in short using meat that is all meat (and lean with it) and other high quality ingredients, has an expensive product on his hands. But as far as taste and texture go, he has no rivals.

With the ever-expanding purchasing power of today's supermarkets, all but the most enterprising independent butchers simply cannot afford to spend time making interesting and original meat products, unless we are prepared to pay extra for them. British meat is very cheap by world standards. In most communities around the world, meat is highly prized; large amounts of it are a luxury. So it is used with care in cooking.

If the nation as a whole wants prime quality lean meat and meat products, we will probably have to be prepared to eat less of it, and pay a higher price per pound. The result would not only be good for the quality of our meals; it would also help to improve our health.

Pies, Sausage Rolls, Luncheon Meats, Pasties, Pâté etc.

Fat, fat and more fat; that's what is in most of these meat products. A pork pie? Three times as much fats as protein. A sausage roll? Five times as much fats as protein. Luncheon meats, pâté, liver sausage, frankfurters, salami? Over three quarters of the calories in these products come from fats, which are mostly 'rubbish' saturated fats. Corned beef is a bit of an exception: half of its calories come from fats. Most meat products are also very salty; they usually contain 2–3 per cent of salt by weight. Salami is 5 per cent salt!

What meat is there in meat products? Usually it is the poorest quality: gristle, sinew, offal, and ground-up unmentionables, re-formed meats, Mechanically Recovered Meat, rind, bone powder, dried blood and plasma, fat – some or all of these things may have found their way into your weekly meat purchases. Another refuse tip for the meat industry, and another good market for the manufacturers of chemical additives.

Why are we so keen on meat products? On the one hand, they are convenient and cheaper than good quality meat. On the other hand, we think of meat as essential to the diet (well, almost everybody who is not a vegetarian does). So we tend to think of meat products as a reasonably nourishing alternative to the joints we can't afford.

As a treat, good quality meat is fine. But most carcass meat in Britain is loaded with saturated fats. The less fatty meat products we eat, the better.

The Compositional Standards for Meat Products

What's in a meat product? Well, according to the new regulations, which came into operation on 12 November 1984 (existing regulations relating to meat products may continue to be complied with until July 1986), the following meat and lean meat contents are laid down by law:

	Minimum meat content (%)	*Minimum lean meat (% of meat content)*
Burger	80	65
Economy Burger	60	65
Hamburger (beef, pork, or beef/pork mixture)	80	65
Chopped X (where X is a specified meat)	90	65
Corned X (where X is a specified meat)	120*	96
Luncheon X (where X is a specified meat)	80	65
Meat Pie / Meat Pudding / Game Pie / Melton Mowbray Pie	cooked 25 / uncooked 21	50 / 50
Scottish Pie	cooked 20 / uncooked 17	50 / 50
Pie / Pudding / Pastie/Pasty / Bridie / Sausage Roll	cooked 12·5 / uncooked 10·5	50 / 50

	Minimum meat content (%)	Minimum lean meat (% of meat content)
Sausage		
Link	pork 65	50
Chipolata	other meat 50	50
Sausage Meat		
Pâté	70	50
Meat Paste	70	65
Spread	70	65

*dehydrated

Anyone interested in further details should consult the regulations in full. They can be obtained from HMSO Bookshops (Statutory Instruments, 1984, No. 1566, *Meat Products and Spreadable Fish Products Regulations*, 1984).

Whereas the Food Standards Committee recommended in 1980 that meat products should in future be labelled with their *lean meat* content, the regulation as of 1984 is that they should be labelled with their *meat* content only: 'minimum x% meat'. There is no maximum fat or water content, except in so far as fat and water are limited by the compositional regulations for meat and lean meat.

In addition to complying with the Meat Products regulations, a manufacturer must also comply with the Food and Drugs Act 1955, the Trade Descriptions Act 1968, and the Food Labelling Regulations 1984. Between them, these say it is an offence to add any substance to food so as to render it injurious to health. It is an offence to sell to the prejudice of the purchaser food which is not of the nature, substance or quality demanded. A manufacturer is not at liberty to use a label or advertisement which falsely describes a food, or misleads as to its nature, substance or quality, including its nutritive or dietary value. It is also an offence to sell food unfit for human consumption. And the food must be labelled with a suitable name, and a list of its ingredients.

If you are not satisfied about the quality of a meat product (or indeed, of any food), ask your Local Authority Trading Standards Officer to investigate. They are there for your benefit, and can help us best if we communicate with them. Their job is to enforce the law. You can contact them via your Town Hall, Shire Hall, or through the Local Authority offices.

What Meat is Best to Eat?

What's the best advice with meats and meat products? A lot of people nowadays don't need much encouragement to become vegetarian, with Prince Charles leading the way. The Vegetarian Society estimates that in 1984 there were 2 million vegetarians and vegans in Britain; and the meat trade is certainly in a bit of a panic. From the health point of view there is almost everything to be said for being vegetarian. If you don't eat meat, and at the same time take some trouble to eat a wide range of cereal and vegetable products, you are likely to become healthier than meat eaters.

Other people don't mind the idea of cutting down on meat and cutting right down on meat products, but are not prepared to go vegetarian. Whether it is steaks, or stews with beef, or salami, there is some kind of meat they won't forego. From the health point of view there is no problem here. If you stop eating any old meat as a routine and instead become a connoisseur of particular high quality or very tasty meats, eating them occasionally, that's fine. Otherwise just eat meat as a relish. Forget the idea that meat should be in the centre of the table and the centre of the plate, in any main meal.

Many other people will always think of themselves as meat-eaters: in a family, husbands more so than wives, perhaps. What then? Well, if you stuff yourself with meat and meat products, you are almost certainly stuffing your arteries with fatty deposits. The right move is to cut down. But also, eat leaner meat: trim fat off meat, eat more poultry, don't fry meat, don't add saturated fats in the cooking of meat. And as always, go for quality. If you are lucky enough to find free-range meat, prefer it and be prepared to pay for the privilege. Once again, cut right down on cheap, convenience meat product foods. You wouldn't feed them to the dog.

The positively good news, for people who like to eat flesh, is that some animal products are positively good for your health. These include game animals and birds: rabbits, hare, deer (venison); pigeon, grouse, pheasant. All of these are seasonal or hard to come by or pricey. Because they are (relatively) wild animals, their flesh has less fat, and what fat they do have is relatively high in healthy polyunsaturates. The strong recommendation is that you do indeed think of fish as the big dish. Fatty fish can be expensive: salmon, trout. But they can be cheap: herring, mackerel, sprats, sardines (from the fishmonger). These cheap sea fish almost vanished from our diet not long ago. The consumption of fatty fish is now a small fraction of what it was at the turn of the century. In times gone by fatty fish was staple food: the wars between England and Holland in the seventeenth century were fought over the herring fishing rights in the North Sea. The message is that the best animal to eat is an animal that, in life, was fit.

Meat: Protein? Or Fat?

Here is a public health warning. When you read that sausages contain around 26 per cent fats (that's around one quarter) you may feel reassured. After all, the NACNE report says that we should cut down our intake of fats to 30 per cent. By this reckoning, sausages sound like reasonably good news. Wrong! There are two totally different ways of measuring the nutrient content of foods, and they are always getting muddled up. The 26 per cent of fats in a sausage, is of *total weight*. The 30 per cent fats recommended is of *total energy* (or calories). If a food is all or almost all fats (butter, for instance, or oils) then these two different methods of measurement add up to much the same figure. But in the case of meat and meat products, there is an enormous difference. For a start, red meat is over half water. Water is heavy but has no energy value. Secondly, almost all the edible parts of meat are made up either of protein or fats – and fats have more than twice the energy of protein, weight for weight.

What this means in practice is that, while 26 per cent of a sausage is fats by weight, the percentage of the energy (calories) in a sausage supplied by fats is 70–80 per cent. However lean the red meat, and however carefully you trim off the visible fat, maybe half its energy will nevertheless come from the fats contained within the meat. If you want to eat protein without fats eat wholemeal bread, beans, lentils and white fish.

The British Government is now considering how to make food labels more helpful to the buyer. We need to know, for all foods, what percentage of fats, saturated fats and sugars and salt they contain.

But the percentage of fats, saturated fats and sugars should be not of total weight, but of total calories. In scientists' terms, the crucial figure is of dry weight, not wet weight. Otherwise we will read that sausages are 26 per cent fats and thus be deceived: for there's no doubt that, given a choice, the sausage manufacturers would rather label by weight (water and all) than by energy. In which case, there would be lies, damned lies – and labels.

Meat and Poultry – A Summary of the Advice

- Choose smaller quantities of leaner cuts of beef, lamb and pork.

- Eat more poultry, game and fish.

- Remove skin from poultry when you cook stews and curries.

- Grill rather than fry.

- Cut off all the visible fat.

- Remove the fat from stews before serving.

- Remove the fat from meat juices before making gravy.

- Buy sausages from a reputable butcher who uses less fatty meat.

- Eat fewer pies. Again, visit a reputable butcher or delicatessen.

- Eat less processed and tinned meats.

- Use more vegetables in cooking.

CHAPTER 3

Fish

FISHY BUSINESS. FINGERING THE FISH.
BATTERED FISH (NON-ACCIDENTAL INJURY).
DOUBLE GLAZING. FISH AND CHIPS.

Animals that are fit and live free are likely to be healthy to eat. Seafood is now the only major part of our diet that has to be hunted. Man has no direct control over the eating habits of ocean fish. They have not been domesticated, enclosed or bred. Their flesh as a result should be healthy to eat, although industrial pollution of course can affect all marine and fresh water life.

How much fish do we eat? One of the largest fish-eating countries in Europe, the UK consumes around 370,000 tonnes, at a retail value of £1.2 billion. This works out at a weekly total of just under 5 oz per person per week, and only 1 oz of it is fresh. All the rest is purchased frozen or processed (mostly canned).

At the beginning of the century, we ate about three times that amount, and in past centuries seafoods such as herring, oysters, salmon, cockles and whelks were staple foods of a huge proportion of the UK population.

Since the Second World War, fresh fish consumption has declined by about 20 per cent. Rising prices, cod wars and overfishing of herring stocks have all taken their toll, and consumers have lost interest.

Fish is poorly advertised. Wet fish shops have all but vanished from many towns. Few of us nowadays have the chance to eat really fresh fish.

And as fast as the wet fish shops have vanished, the frozen fish and fish product industries have been busying themselves with new processing techniques.

Fishy Business

Some very peculiar things have been going on in the fish processing industry in the last few years. You might perhaps suppose that a cod or a prawn is not a thing that can be much tampered with before it reaches the supermarket freezer or fishmonger's slab. Indeed many of those people and organizations whose job it is to safeguard consumers' interests, have shown a surprising lack of interest in the procedures which have been going on behind the doors of fish factories in the last decade.

However in 1984, all that changed. A most interesting report was published by the Institute of Trading Standards Administration, entitled *Fish Technology – its Uses and Abuses*. This report by David Walker (Trading Standards Officer for Shropshire County Council) described in detail how and why the quality of fish and fish products has deteriorated over the years. The disappearing fish finger, the water-logged fillet, double glazed prawns, minced bones, 'frame' mince, reformed scampi, vegetable protein 'extenders', emulsifying agents, simulated salmon – these and other wondrous developments have been carefully investigated and described. The report has now been taken up by the Food Advisory Committee of the Ministry of Agriculture, the committee which advises government on legislation concerning food quality and labelling. Here are some of the main findings of the report.

Fish Blocks

The cod war and the extension of national fishing limits to 200 miles effectively wrecked the UK deep-sea trawling industry, which had at its peak about 50 ships, but was reduced to 10–15 trawlers by 1982. The steep decline in the amount of white fish landed left a hole in the market, so that we now import some 65 per cent of all the cod we eat. And herein lies a problem. For much of this fish arrives in Britain in the form of fish blocks which are later carved up to create fish fingers, breaded fish pieces and other products. It is the method of construction of these blocks which gives rise for concern.

How does white fish come to be squeezed and moulded into a standard sized block? The fish are filleted, by hand or machine, packed into a mould, and frozen. Freezing causes fish to expand, thus the fish fill the mould. Nothing wrong with that surely?

No, nothing wrong with it, provided that the final block is what it should be, fish and fish alone. The trouble is that the temptation to add a little something to spin out an expensive raw material is sometimes just too great. After all, water has done wonders for the meat processing industry; why shouldn't it do the same for the fish processors? What has been happening is that the manufacturers of the blocks have found that sodium polyphosphate does wonders for a fillet. Spray or drip fish into polyphosphate solution, or put the two together into what looks like a builder's concrete mixer for a little tumble, and out comes a nicely expanded fish!

And naturally, the leading lights of the polyphosphate fish movement are only too eager to describe the immense advantages to us, the consumers. Their arguments are strangely familiar: it improves the texture, improves appearance, reduces 'drip loss' on thawing, helps in making proper blocks with nice sharp edges that cut smoothly. Heard it all before? Well, something like it anyway, from the specialists in tumbling and massaging and expanding meat.

Not everyone involved in the production of fish blocks goes

in for such practices. And many manufacturers of fish fingers and breaded fish products go to great lengths to ensure that they are buying fish and fish alone. But because many of the blocks are imported, it is a difficult business to ensure good quality. The importance of proper surveillance becomes only too apparent when you realize that up to £6 million worth (or 2400 tonnes) of 'added water' is sold each year in the UK under the guise of 'fish', in fish fingers alone. And we, of course, pay for it.

Minced Fish

What happens to the bits of fish left on the bone after it has been filleted? Until some cunning machinery was invented, much of it was wasted. Now the fish skeletons (or 'frames' as they are known in the trade) and odd bits and pieces, are fed into a bone-separating machine to produce 'fish mince'. The quality of the mince depends on the starting material. Obviously fish fillets would produce the best mince, and pure bones and innards the worst. As with the modern sausage, the aim to use all edible parts of an animal rather than waste them is of course admirable, and fish mince can be made into blocks whose market value is just half as much as those constructed of fillets. But this process is not without its problems. First, fish mince tastes funny. A fish mince block is to fish as chipboard is to wood, and the similarity does not end there, because fish mince can taste like cardboard. It is also tough. The disintegration of tissues releases substances which speed up rancidity, so its storage life is reduced. Minced bones make it taste gritty. And the more bone, blood and entrail present, the greyer the final product. And last, but by no means least, fish mince is the dried pork rind of the fish industry – it sucks up its own weight in water, and that's without any added polyphosphates!

Fish mince is often used in block manufacture, either by itself, or together with fish fillets. In a mixed block, the mince and fillets often go in for an intimate polyphosphate tumble before being cosily packed into moulds. These blocks are then chopped up for fish fingers and other coated products.

The consumer's problem is, once again, how do you know if a fish finger or a breaded fish 'fillet' is the real thing, or a well tumbled and massaged mess of fish mince and water? And if water has been added, how much? And how can you compare the price of a battered cod portion with water, and one without?

Fingering the Fish

Before the 1970s fish fingers were normally made of filleted fish, according to the original American recipe of the 1950s. Invented in the USA in 1952, they were an instant success, as they were on introduction to the UK in 1955. Given that they are almost universally popular with children, and that we spend £100 million buying 40,000 tonnes of them each year, what of their quality today?

The quantity and proportion of fish in a fish finger is a frequent subject of discussion between trading standards officers and the manufacturers. There are no compositional regulations for the minimum fish content of a fish finger (nor, for that matter, are there any for any other breaded or battered fish products), so the consumer is not protected.

How is the fish finger made? Fish blocks are sawn into finger shapes, coated in batter, and covered with breadcrumbs. The finger is partially fried and frozen. Now if you were a fish finger manufacturer and had costs on your mind, you might do what some UK manufacturers have been up to since the early 1970s: choose a cheaper fish block, cut the fingers thinner, spread the batter thicker, add more breadcrumbs. The ratio of fish to coating is an all-important sum which you would be keen to do at frequent intervals. For a thick fish finger has proportionately less batter and crumbs, and more fish, than a thin one. The thinner the finger, the greater the weight of cheap batter you can sell to an unsuspecting customer.

Trading standards officers stated in 1983 that the lean fish content of fish fingers has fallen from 80 per cent in the 1960s, to a present average level of 56 per cent, with a substantial proportion of them also containing added water. Their 1983 analyses of 475 samples (involving 6,500 fish fingers) showed that the lowest quantity of fish was 33.7 per cent, and 13 per cent of fish fingers contained less than half lean fish. Ten per cent of the samples contained more than a fifth added water. Three quarters contained more than a tenth added water. The average was 13.8 per cent. The trading standards officers considered that legislation is urgently needed to control both quality and labelling.

The industry, for their part, maintains that variations in fish content are due to variations in the quality of raw materials, and inadequacy of the chemical test for 'fish', the extra water is in the batter, not the fish, the quality of starting materials is kept at a premium, and, perhaps most important of all, fish fingers have never had a fish content of 80 per cent, so how could it have decreased to the extent maintained by the trading standards officers?

The enforcement officers have conducted many analyses of fish fingers over the years, and while some argument about the methods of analysis may be justified, there can be no doubt that, at the lower end of the market, a very poor quality product is being sold, and that over all, the amount of fish has gone down, and the amount of water and batter, up.

The fish finger of the 1980s is pointing firmly downwards, towards the general debasement of a popular food. It is time that the Ministry of Agriculture's Food Advisory Committee sat down to look at the problem.

Battered Fish (Non-accidental Injury)

Apart from the battering on the outside, there is ample evidence that a lot of coated fish products have been well and truly battered on the inside. 'Reformed' fish, in other words unrecognizable bits of fish stuck together with a liberal dose of polyphosphates, and moulded with great artistry into fillet shapes, are covered with breadcrumbs or batter. Some manufacturers even have the nerve to call these things fish 'fillets'.

Of course, some manufacturers and retailers take great care to ensure that their products are what they say on the label. But once a leading retailer places an enormous order with a manufacturer whose standards are not of the highest quality, it forces others to debase their product in order to compete with a lower price. And with only a handful of supermarkets now accounting for three quarters of the UK grocery trade, competition for these bulk orders is obviously fierce.

Reformed Scampi

Second cousin to the reformed joint of ham, scampi has not escaped the water-holding agents either. Much loved by the catering trade for its ease of preparation, and by the public for its connections with high society, the watered down, reformed, heavily breaded fried scampi is a well-researched animal.

It starts its life as a nice little lobster, whose tail is much in demand. Chopped off, the tail is iced and frozen, whereupon the meat inside expands and cracks the shell. After thawing and shelling, the tails more often than not come to rest in a tankful of polyphosphate solution (what would the food industry do without this helpful chemical?), after which they are extruded, moulded, frozen and coated.

Now any idea you might have had about scampi being a plain ordinary fat shellfish surrounded only in tasty breadcrumbs is quite wrong. For the majority of scampi caught nowadays are miserable little lobsters, caught before they have fully grown. But the bigger the tails, the higher the price. The imaginative manufacturer is not deterred by such a trivial problem as minuscule scampi. The answer is simply to bung them all into a mincer or chopper, mash them together with a good dose of polyphosphates, squeeze it all through a nozzle, and out comes a whopping great scampi all set to attract a premium price!

So, once again, how can you tell the difference between, first, a proper scampi tail; second, one with water added; third, the perfectly formed, watered, polyphosphated article? Is there a price difference? Not necessarily. Does the label say? Hardly ever. Does the restaurant menu give you a clue? Unlikely.

And lest you should think that the only problem is on the inside of a scampi, spare a thought for the amount of breadcrumb on the outsides. Just like the fish finger, the inside is more expensive than the outside. A voluntary Code of Practice says that the scampi content should not be less than 50%. However, if water is added to the scampi before weighing, the Code can clearly be bent. And thick breadcrumbs on a small scampi produce a more profitable article. So the next time you think of buying some scampi for dinner, you might like to ask the supermarket manager or the restaurateur just how much he or she knows about the fish content and composition. You might even decide that real unbattered shellfish are a better choice.

Double Glazing

Beware the double glazing salesman.

Beware the double glazed prawn.

Most of the prawns eaten in the UK are imported, although some are caught in the North Sea. Many are brought into the UK in bulk, and then packed for distribution.

The prawn is cooked, shelled, washed, soaked in brine, frozen and glazed with a very thin coating of ice, which protects the prawn during storage. The weight of glaze comes to about a tenth of the final weight of the prawn, if the process is done with care. However, unscrupulous processors manage to add up to a third by weight of ice, and the worst of all import already glazed prawns, and give them another going over before packing and sale!

A survey of prawns and their prices revealed an average glaze content of a quarter, with a range in price of £1.99 to £4.78 per pound. 'The consumer would appear to be paying on average something in the region of 63p per pack for the privilege of purchasing iced water.' In his report, the Trading Standards Officer for Shropshire then estimates that 'if only a tenth of glaze was applied to prawns imported into the UK from one country alone, it would amount to an annual sale of some 660 tonnes of iced water at a prawn price of over £4 million'. (And that tenth is a very conservative estimate.)

This outrageous and possibly fraudulent practice is, of course, not common to all prawn wholesalers. But how is the honest salesman to keep his share of the market while others go in for such profiteering and dishonest methods which go largely undetected by the general public?

Fish – Wetter Than Wet

Lest you are by this stage beginning to glaze over at the thought of yet more water, more polyphosphates, more lost money, stop and think about what a nice coating of ice glaze can do for the appearance and appeal of a fillet of cod or plaice, or even for a whole 'fresh' fish. Without glaze, white fish is apparently all right when fresh, but pretty nasty when frozen and then thawed. Its skin is dull, yellowish, flaccid. Delicately glazed with polyphosphates and water, it is restored to its former beauty; shining, full blue-white and appetizing.

The glaze is applied by spray, or by dipping the fish into water prior to freezing. And the problem for the consumer is that the fish is weighed after glazing, not before! As with the batter on a fish finger, a flat, thin fish like plaice picks up more glaze than round, solid ones like cod. And once again, we, the public pay for the water, in this case about a twentieth by weight, which works out at a market value of around £4·8 million per year.

The Ministry of Agriculture Food Standards Committee recommended in 1978 that glazed fish should be labelled as such. Once again, the recommendation has not been adopted. Once again, the consumer loses out.

Fishing For Quality

Faced with all these problems, how can you be sure you are getting value for money, and a fish that tastes as it should?

Now that wet fish shops have become a rare sight in our high streets, big supermarkets have taken an interest, and are setting up fresh fish counters. Some even tell you how to cook your dinner, because they realize that the nation as a whole has long forgotten what to do with a piece of cod other than shove it in the frying pan.

Cod, plaice, haddock, whiting – these are the fish we usually eat. Yet there are many others that most of us have probably never tried. Visit your local fishmonger, if you have one. Ask if you see a strange looking fish, and how to cook it.

But first, be sure you know what really fresh fish looks like. A bright eye, red shining gills, a mildly seaweedy smell and firm flesh indicate that the fish is fresh. By contrast, fish is stale when the eye is sunken and opaque, when the flesh is soft to touch and remains indented if you prod it with your finger, and the skin is dry and gritty or starting to look slimy. And of course, you can tell stale fish by the smell.

Get to know your fishmongers. Tell them if you are not satisfied and they will know which wholesaler to avoid in future. Only with better communication will our supplies of fish improve. And with luck, fishmongers will introduce us to new fish and different ways of cooking them.

The first thing you need to know is how to clean fresh fish, because, although the fishmonger should do it for you, a few fish arrive home with their innards intact. The longer the intestines stay inside the fish, the faster it will deteriorate because of the bacteria. Cut off the fins, scrape the scales off by drawing a blunt knife underneath from back to front. Take out the intestines by slitting the fish up the belly, or cutting through the gills. The liver and the roes may be good to eat. Wash the fish under cold water.

Most 'fresh' fish in Britain has actually been frozen before it comes to rest on the fishmonger's slab. Almost none of it is fished out of the sea in nets, into the bottom of a boat, put on to lorries and delivered for sale within 24 hours. To eat fish that is truly fresh, you will have to visit the remaining fishermen in the coastal towns and villages, and the few inland fishmongers who guarantee a really fresh product. Local fish is often sold with just that written on the label: 'local fish'.

The rest of Britain's 'fresh' fish comes to market frozen from British and foreign deep-sea trawlers that put out to sea for days at a time. Trawler fishing developed in the second half of the nineteenth century after ice-making machinery had been invented. Before that, ice had to be transported from Iceland.

The nation's taste for white fish developed after steam trawlers went to work in the 1860s and 1870s in the North Sea. The fish was frozen on board, packed in ice and despatched by rail to inland towns on the same day. This meant that the majority of the inland population of Britain could buy really white fresh fish for the first time. Before then, only salted and pickled herrings were usually available to the working classes.

White Fish

White fish are just what the name implies – white cod, haddock, whiting, plaice, skate, hake, flounder, dab, halibut, turbot, sole, brill . . . There are so many delicious fish that most of us have never tasted.

All white fish contain good quality protein, vitamins and minerals, which is why they are an important part of a healthy diet rather than fatty red meat and meat products.

Fatty Fish

Eel, sprats, herring, bloater, mackerel, pilchard, salmon, sardine, tuna, trout: all these fish have fatty flesh.

Fish are cold blooded. In other words, they adopt the temperature of their environment. Sea water, and particularly the North Sea, tends to be a bit chilly, so the fish swimming in it are cold inside. What would happen if, like butter, the fat inside the muscle of a fish were solid at North Sea temperatures? Herring might have a bit of trouble swimming along with a tail of freezing, lard-like consistency. Fish fat is so high in polyunsaturates that it stays liquid even at North Sea temperatures. Fish fat is very different from meat fat.

This sort of fat is very beneficial, and can help to prevent heart attacks and strokes. There is a good deal of interest in one particular fish fat, eicosapentaenoic acid (EPA), which is known to reduce blood viscosity as well as reducing its stickiness. New research suggests that a high-fish diet may possibly help to prevent multiple sclerosis and also rheumatoid arthritis, and also to relieve the symptoms of these crippling diseases. So, although the general advice is to eat less fats, fish fat in particular is healthy. And fresh, fatty fish is best because smoked fish is very salty.

Shellfish

Several years ago people began to worry about shellfish, because it was said they contained a lot of cholesterol. But eating shellfish is very unlikely to increase your blood cholesterol dramatically. For a start, most of us eat hardly any shellfish. The average consumption is 0·09 oz per head per week. Secondly, the indications are that the cholesterol-like compound in shellfish probably has no harmful effects. Thirdly, shellfish are often eaten in large quantities in countries where rates of heart disease are low.

Crabs, lobsters, prawns, shrimps, mussels, crayfish, oysters, clams, scallops, sea urchins – many of them are rare and expensive. But before you reject them, how much does your Sunday lunch cost? Not all of us can afford roast beef, but all the same many families spend a lot of money on meat each week. Why not have some interesting shellfish instead on occasions? Ask your friends or the fishmonger how to cook shellfish if you are not sure. Buy them from a reputable shop, and beware the double glazing!

Freshwater Fish

Inland fish farming is beginning to make quite a big contribution to fish sales. Freshwater trout must be completely fresh, otherwise their flavour tends to become quickly tainted. If trout from a trout farm has a strong 'earthy' flavour, tell the fishmonger. The farm should change the water.

Like all fatty fish, both trout and eels are high in polyunsaturated fats. Fresh eels are delicious but difficult to find.

Cooking Fish

Too often, fish are flung into the frying pan with butter, sprinkled with salt and dumped beside a pile of chips. The goodness of fish is all but ruined once the butter has soaked in. Is there no better, healthier way of cooking them?

If you really like fried fish, use oil instead of butter. But try new methods as well. Fish is delicious baked in the oven with herbs or onions. It can be steamed with spices and onions Chinese style, or grilled. Mackerel and sprats are very good grilled with a little French mustard.

Does fish always need salt? If you use no other flavouring, you will probably resort to the salt-pot. But lemon, parsley, dill, fennel – so many herbs are good with fish. Why cover the flavour with salt?

Fish and Chips

Fish and chips were invented in the 1860s, and only became popular when the price of fish fell as new deep-sea trawlers started to bring back large quantities of cod from northern waters. Fish and chips were the invention of the working classes, and were popular by the start of the First World War.

Traditionally fish and chips have always been fried in lard and hard fats. The changeover to vegetable oils has happened sooner in the south than in the north. Most deep-fryers are now filled with groundnut oil, blended vegetable oil, or hard vegetable fats. Of these, groundnut oil is the most expensive, and is regarded by those in the business as the best because it does not burn. Vegetable oil, on the other hand, quickly produces charred bits and pieces, and according to chip shop owners in London's East End, soaks into the chips making them 'real disgustin'. And the blocks of hardened vegetable fats, or palm oil, are of course highly saturated.

Groundnut oil is fairly low in saturated fats, whereas blended vegetable oil is anybody's guess. Repeated heating and cooling of oils can make them more saturated, and there have been worries that harmful chemicals can build up in the oil from overheated residues. But if the chip shop has a high turnover, and is frying almost continuously, then the water vapour produced by the frying chips forms a layer over the top of the oil which prevents the polyunsaturates being oxidized, or changed, by the air into more saturated fats. And a shop with a high turnover will have to top up the oil quite frequently, so the oil is fresher.

Furthermore if the oil is carefully and regularly filtered to remove burnt residues, then the chips could be altogether rather a healthy affair. But before you rush off for a large bagful, you might like to ask the chip shop owner a few questions: what kind of oil does the shop use? How saturated is it? How many preservatives and other additives does it contain? Which ones? How long has it been in the pan? Analysis of chip shop oils has shown enormous variation in the saturated fat content.

Fish and chips can be an extremely fatty meal. Much depends on the quality of the potatoes. Floury potatoes soak up more fats than hard, crisp varieties. Big chips soak up less fats than little ones (their surface area is smaller). The fattiest chips of all are those that are reconstituted from potato starch. The potatoes are pulped and the starch squeezed through a chip machine. You can tell the chips that have been produced like this because they are all exactly the same diameter, often with wavy edges. A hardened chip-eater knows the difference, and knows where to find the real thing.

Deep-fried food is all right to eat occasionally. It is not all right to have every day, or even every other day, if the fat is very saturated. People who run fish and chips shops and other take-aways, and canteen managers, should be made aware of the harm they do to their customers if the fats they use are saturated and if they do not clean out their pans often enough. And lest you think that the fat is the only problem with fish and chips, you might be interested to know that a curious development took place in the flavouring industry many years ago. For brown vinegar has often been replaced by a by-product of the petroleum industry! The brown stuff that is sprinkled in your bag of chips may not be what you had bargained for.

Fish Fingers and Fishcakes

Many children love fish fingers and fishcakes, and they are easy to cook. Grill them rather than fry. If your children are in the habit of having them fried, use a good oil. Fish fingers are much healthier than sausages, processed meats and hamburgers, although the larger the quantity of batter, the larger the amount of saturated fat the fish finger is likely to contain. (Batter consists chiefly of crumbs and fat.) The original recipe for fish fingers was a good example of useful food-processing. However, why do many fish fingers and fish cakes now sold in Britain have to be the colour of marigolds? Their yellow colouring is often a coal tar dye, tartrazine (E102), that, like all coal tar dyes, can prove to be carcinogenic, and known to cause allergic reactions in sensitive individuals, notably children.

Tinned Fish

'Sardines in edible oil':

Does that strike you as being rather a curious thing to write on a tin of food? Edible is surely the very least that one would expect. What else could it be? Engine oil? Paraquat?

It is a perfect example of a completely useless food label. All of us expect food to be edible. Even if you don't drink the oil, you'll be eating the sardines that were swimming in it.

What would be far more helpful would be some more detailed information about that oil – information that would tell us not that it is edible, but whether it is good to eat, which is rather a different thing. Healthy fish can swim in unhealthy oil, saturated with salt.

Look for sardines in named oils. The 'vegetable oils' or plain 'oils' frequently used may in fact be quite harmless (for example soya oil). But unless they tell you, how can you know?

Tinned fish is a better nutritional bet than many tinned and processed meats. Both contain too much salt, but the fish is likely to contain little saturated fats, even when in oil.

Fish – A Summary of the Advice

- Eat more fresh fish of all kinds, white and fatty.
- Cook fish with less butter. Use oils instead.
- Try more herbs, spices, lemon juice instead of salt.
- Avoid ready prepared fish dishes in fatty sauces.
- Fish fingers are better than sausages and hamburgers!

CHAPTER 4

Bread and Cereals

THE RELEGATION OF BREAD. BREAD DOESN'T MAKE YOU FAT.
GRINDING AWAY THE GOODNESS. WHOLEMEAL: THE STAFF OF LIFE.

The cultivation of rice, barley, oats, wheat, millet, rye and corn (maize) transformed human society from 'hunter and gatherer' to settled agriculturist. These crops, developed from wild grasses, became staple foods of civilization around the world. It is only during the twentieth century that the most industrialized nations have started to eat less of them in favour of more expensive meats, dairy foods and eggs. The British now generally regard cereals, fruits and vegetables as inferior to animal foods. Yet we are putting our health at risk by eating too little of them.

We eat too many fats and sugars, and not enough wholegrain cereals. Wholegrain cereals are those that arrive on your plate intact, with their outer fibrous coat of bran. It has not been removed by milling. Wheat, maize, millets, barley, oats, rye and rice can all be eaten as whole grains. They can be prepared either as the grain itself, or ground into flour to make bread, pancakes, biscuits, cakes etc.

At the very least the lack of these whole foods causes serious intestinal problems. Wholegrain cereals and starchy vegetables are healthy. They are not fattening, and avoiding them is not the right way to lose weight.

The Relegation of Bread

For most of the twentieth century, the British population has been instructed that starchy carbohydrate foods such as bread and potatoes are quite inferior to animal products, and that a more meaty, milky diet is the healthiest way to proceed. This message has pervaded our whole economy, to the extent that since the 1930s great efforts have been made to increase dairy and meat production. The aim was to have every man, woman and child drinking 1 pint of milk per day. This target has never been reached.

Bread and potatoes were considered 'energy' food in contrast with meat, milk, eggs, cheese etc, which were 'protein' foods. The national diet was neatly divided into groups:

'energy' foods	*'growth' foods*
(fats and carbohydrates)	(protein)
bread, potatoes,	meat, milk,
fats, oils, sugars	cheese, eggs, fish, beans

'protective' foods
(minerals and vitamins)
fresh fruit, fresh vegetables,
meat, bread, milk

These groups found their way into doctors' waiting-rooms throughout the land. They were taught in schools and universities, in domestic science classes, in cookery books. Protein was good because it was essential for growth and repair of body tissues. Protective foods were good because they fought off infections, kept the system running smoothly. Energy foods were all right provided you did not eat more than you needed to keep up all your energy and vitality and maintain body weight.

The classification did not stop there. Years and years of research into the quality of different sorts of proteins led to the high protein foods being further sub-divided into first- and second-class. First-class were meats, fish, milk and eggs, because they were closest in value to human breast milk, which produces optimal growth in babies. Second-class were bread and beans, because they were not quite so good as breast milk and eggs.

So bread and potatoes were second-best. The attitude was that they might have the odd vitamin and second-class protein, but in the main they were good for one thing only – energy. And that is how they were described to the population.

That said, the doctors and nutritionists who did the research and drew the conclusions were working in a rather different situation from today. In the late nineteenth and first half of the twentieth centuries, very large numbers of people suffered from chronic under-nutrition. Many nutritionists had a strong commitment to social change. Their observations showed that the mass of the population was in very poor shape, suffering from vitamin, energy and protein deficiencies. Scientists thought animal proteins had superior properties to those of plants, and therefore their consumption was encouraged. In addition scientists believed from their research on animal growth that large amounts of protein were needed. We now know this is wrong.

The general nutrition of the population was definitely substandard. Rationing in the Second World War provided nutritionists with their first real opportunity to ensure that everyone received a fair share of the nation's larder, and a healthy diet. The weekly ration in the Second World War consisted of 4 oz of bacon and ham, 3 oz of cheese, 8 oz of sugar, 4 oz of preserves, 8 oz of fats and 1s 2d worth of meat (amounting to a few ounces). The population filled themselves up on bread and potatoes, which were not rationed. This was a low-fats, low-sugars, high fibre and high starch diet. The health of the mass of the population had never been so good.

During and after the war nutrition education was part of government policy. The food groups – proteins, energy, protective foods – were taught vigorously throughout the country. The message stuck then, and it is still firmly stuck in the public mind: bread and potatoes are second-class food.

A further influence was the widespread publicity given to low carbohydrate diets for weight loss. This still continues. Stationery and book shops throughout the land abound with paperback diet books telling you to avoid bread, potatoes, pasta, rice. Anything with carbohydrate in it must be shunned like the plague.

All the while these nutrition messages were finding their way into the public mind, and sticking there, a few single-minded doctors and scientists were having serious misgivings about it all. First there was Dr Thomas Allinson in the nineteenth century, convinced of the value of wholemeal bread. Then there was Sir Robert McCarrison, whose work in India convinced him that the rich, over-refined diet being advocated in the West was distinctly inferior to that of the poorer peasant communities in India. Dental decay, obesity, coronary heart disease, constipation, piles, cancer – these and other problems were thought by McCarrison to be caused by over-refined foods. His work led to the foundation of the McCarrison Society, devoted today to the improvement of British eating habits. Then there was the British naval Surgeon-Captain T. L. Cleave, who died in 1983. His thesis was that Western illnesses are caused by eating too much refined sugar and not enough whole grain cereals. His ideas were taken up by Dr Hugh Trowell and Dr Denis Burkitt, leading figures in advocating further research into the effects of wholegrain foods on human metabolism. The results of research that they have stimulated suggest that they were absolutely right. We eat far too few wholegrain cereals, fruit and vegetables, and too much in the way of refined sugars.

Starch and Fibre – What Do They Do?

Starches and sugars should no longer be grouped together as carbohydrates with similar values, as we have all been taught.

Carbohydrate is simply the general name given to a whole range of different compounds found in large quantities in plant, and also in animal foods. Starches, sugars and dietary fibre are all carbohydrates, but by no means are they all the same. (Sugars are dealt with in Chapter 9.)

Starch can be refined in just the same way as sugar. In other words it is separated from its parent plant and processed into pure starch. Cornflour is a good example of a refined starch – it is separated from the rest of the corn grain in the same way that sugar is separated from the sugar cane and sugar beet. White household, plain flour has been separated from the outer part of the wheat grain during grinding.

It is this separation of starch from the rest of the nutritious, fibrous plant material that is harmful. The shops are full of foods that are made in this way: potato and corn starch turned into crunchy snacks, cakes and biscuits made with white flour, sauces made with starch, refined starch in sausages and meat pies, white flour in pastries. All these foods and many, many more are made with starch that has been separated from most of its dietary fibre.

Dietary fibre is the fibrous bit of a plant. The outer fibrous coat of a grain is called bran. Wheat, barley, oats, rye, maize, rice – all these grains in their unrefined state consist of a starchy middle and a fibrous bran coat. For health we need more wholegrain cereals, and fewer refined starches.

Dietary fibre does several things. First, it makes food travel faster through your intestine. Second, it makes your stools softer, preventing constipation and damage to the walls of the intestine. Third, because it encourages speed in the lower regions, it is thought to prevent toxic chemicals lurking around next to your intestinal wall and causing damage. Fourth, it may actually produce beneficial changes in places other than the intestine, such as the blood stream. Fifth, it helps to prevent tooth decay. A tablespoon of sugar provides the perfect food for bacteria in your mouth to set to work on. A tablespoon of sugar cane would give them practically nothing, because the tiny amount of sugar it contains is so diluted by water and fibrous material. The bacteria would have to munch their way through the cane fibre before they got to the sugar. A small piece of cane residue between the teeth provides almost nothing for the bacteria, whereas a small residue of that tablespoon of sugar is good concentrated food for them.

Refined starch, eaten without its dietary fibre, and in association with refined sugars, also rots the teeth and it constipates. Food travels slowly through the intestine, the faeces become small, hard and impacted. Their owner reaches for the laxatives and visits the dentist.

Many illnesses caused by lack of dietary fibre do not become clinically important until adult life; in other words, you get no symptoms in childhood and early adulthood. Children do not often complain of constipation, but constipated many of them undoubtedly are. The serious discomfort that constipation causes in adult life is probably the result of a continually constipated childhood – bunged-up for life. Diverticular disease, the development of abnormal little pockets in the intestine, can be very painful and serious in adulthood, but is rare in children. It is most probably caused by life-long constipation. So are piles or haemorrhoids (varicose veins in the anal canal). And colon cancer is probably, in part, caused by lack of dietary fibre.

Bread Doesn't Make You Fat

Avoiding starchy foods is not the answer to the problem of overweight. On the contrary, if you are overweight, you should eat more starchy foods.

Eating a lot of calorie-heavy foods is one of the causes of overweight, and fats are the most fattening of all the foods we eat. Butter provides 740 calories per 100 grams (about 3½ oz). The same amount of bread provides 216 calories, and 100 grams of potatoes provides only 87 calories. Fats are the most calorie-heavy foods in our diets.

Then there is the effect removing the fibre, or refining the starches and sugars, has on the quantity of food you can eat. It is easy to eat a teaspoon of sugar. But how long would it take you to munch your way through the large sugar beet from which it was refined? A tablespoon of starch and sugar which arrives on your plate complete with its accompanying dietary fibre is considerably bulkier than the refined (separated) equivalent. You simply cannot eat as much.

Obesity can be corrected in two ways. First, by avoiding sugars, in all their forms, eating less fats, particularly saturated fats, and drinking less alcohol. And, second, by increasing physical activity.

BREAD: THE STAFF OF LIFE?

Which breads should you choose? Is brown the same as wholemeal? What are Granary and Hovis? How can you tell which is which?

The whole wheat grain consists of an outer fibrous bran layer, the germ (the embryo from which a new plant would grow) and the inner white endosperm. The bran contains the fibre and protein, the germ contains most of the minerals, protein, vitamins and oils, and the endosperm contains starch and protein.

When wholewheat grains are ground to make flour, this is what happens.

Nearly all flour in Britain is ground up between steel rollers. It passes through twenty or thirty sets of rollers, sifters and 'purifiers'. The bran is the first to be separated from the grain, then the germ, then the starchy inside. The millers collect all these streams separately – a pile of bran, a pile of germ and a pile of white endosperm plus some intermediate piles. From these piles, flours of different degrees of brownness and whiteness are created.

If you ground your own wheat grains in a coffee grinder, you would be quite sure that the resulting flour would contain all the bits of wheat. You could see that none of it had been removed. It would be 100 per cent whole wheat.

Wholemeal flour produced in roller mills can be a bit different. Who knows if the bits of white, the bran and the germ have been recombined in the right proportions? In other words, if the miller puts some of the white flour into a sack, and then some bran, and only a minute amount of the germ, who will know?

But will the flour be wholemeal? This is just what happens in some mills. The different streams are put back together to make brown and wholemeal flour. Recombining the different 'streams' produces breads with different amounts of fibre, and this is the reason why we, the consumers, do not know exactly how much fibre there is in our bread, or, indeed, how much wheatgerm.

There are differences in the quality of different wholemeal breads, of which more later. But there are also distinct and important differences between white, brown (wheatmeal), Granary, Hovis and wholemeal.

White Bread: A National Disgrace

White flour, and the white bread made from it, is 72 per cent extraction. That is, the flour is composed of the inside 72 per cent of the grain. The outer 28 per cent, which contains almost all the germ and the bran, has been removed during milling. Therefore white flour and white bread are almost entirely endosperm – starch and protein. They contain less than one third of the fibre in wholemeal flour, and a good deal less of the minerals and vitamins.

During milling to produce white flour, the vitamin, mineral and essential fats content of the grain is reduced dramatically, because they are nearly all in the bran and germ. The government therefore requires millers to put back two B vitamins, plus iron and calcium. The B vitamins and iron must be partially restored to the level of 85 per cent extraction flour.

Calcium is added, in abundance, as chalk (it's quite a lot cheaper than flour!). Wholemeal flour contains 35 mg calcium per 100 grams. As a result of fortification with chalk, white flour contains 140 mg calcium per 100 grams, four times as much.

The government has recently decided not to follow the advice of a Department of Health COMA expert committee that reported on bread and flour. This committee recommended the repeal of the regulations. If this had happened, the two B vitamins, iron and calcium, would no longer have had to be added to white bread. But if bread were not fortified with vitamin B_1 (thiamine) and calcium large numbers of people, particularly the poor and elderly, and women, would be lacking. Vitamin B_1 deficiency causes depression, irritability, weakness and loss of weight. Calcium deficiency causes anaemia, and weakness in the bones and teeth.

When white flour is used to make white bread, it is not just wheat and yeast that go into the mixer. Dozens of additives are permitted in white and brown breads. Some, like vitamin C, are harmless. The effect of some others is unknown. Others are 'anti-nutrients'. These certainly do the body no good, and may damage the health of vulnerable people.

The reason why all these chemicals are added is to help manufacturers' machinery to produce a uniform product of high volume and keeping quality. White bread is made by the highly mechanized Chorleywood Bread Process. White flour is mixed at tremendously high speed with a potent brew of water, yeast, sugar, salt, yeast nutrients, chemical improvers, fats and several other goodies, which have the combined effect of doing away with the hours of fermentation traditional bread-making requires. This is why Chorleywood bread is so tasteless. There is no time for the yeast to get to work on the dough. It is mixed, risen and baked to produce a loaf containing more water and more air than you could ever create successfully in your own kitchen.

White, sliced, plastic wrapped bread is a disgraceful product, of which the nation should be ashamed. Why otherwise does the British public go on and on about how wonderful French bread is? You can bet your boots that the heads of research at big bakeries do not usually eat it!

So why do we eat it? Because it is cheaper than any other kind of bread. The big baker/miller conglomerates, having invested vast sums in machinery to mill white flour to produce white bread, are so desperate to sell their product to the public that they are prepared to give huge discounts to the supermarkets in order to guarantee a sale. They make their bread the cheapest available. This is not to say that those who work in these bread factories are all bent on the destruction of our intestines, but that, faced with years of capital investment in machinery, they have no choice but to use every method within their power to make their products sell. And the master bakers, who buy their flour at prices set by the big miller/baker conglomerates, simply cannot afford to sell their bread at such low prices.

And it is not only the white sliced article that is of such poor quality. The vast majority of British bread is made in a similar way, even in the master bakers' ovens. They also use a short fermentation, speeded along with chemical improvers. Their white bread is often no better than the plastic-wrapped variety.

It is no surprise that sales of white bread have been dropping ever since the 1950s. Now, sales of brown and wholemeal are still small, but they are increasing, and not just among the middle classes. But do you know which is which among the browns, Granaries, Hovis and wholemeals?

Brown – Not the Real Thing

Brown bread is sometimes called 'wheatmeal', although proposed legislation will do away with this meaningless term. Brown bread usually consists of 85 per cent extraction flour – in other words, flour containing the inner 85 per cent of the whole grain. The outer 15 per cent has been removed. It follows therefore, that brown is not wholemeal. This may be news to some readers, and even to some sales assistants in bakeries, who often do not seem to understand the difference between brown and wholemeal.

Brown bread contains more bran than white bread, and it should contain more germ. Therefore it has higher mineral, vitamin and fibre levels. However, when the big millers make brown flour from their 'streams' of wheat, they do not always put the germ back. Sometimes only white flour and bran go into the sack.

Brown bread can be made with the same chemical improvers, antioxidants, anti-stalers etc. as white bread. It also has one other useful additive – useful, that is, to the manufacturers – caramel. Caramel colouring makes you think the bread is browner than it really is. If you usually eat this brown bread, buy a loaf of wholemeal and compare the colour. Take a good look at the closeness of the grain, at the size of the bits of bran. The well trained eye can detect a dyed brown loaf at one glance.

Brown bread can be made using the Chorleywood Bread Process, just like white. So again, there is no long fermentation process to enhance the flavour, and again you are presented with wet, aerated bread. Sub-standard again, both in baking quality and nutritional value. But brown bread is better than white. If the entire population changed tomorrow from their predominantly white bread diet to brown, their health would undoubtedly improve.

Granary bread is an interesting mixture. Officially, it is the trade mark owned by Rank Hovis for a particular bread recipe. The name granary can mean many things. According to Rank Hovis, their Granary is wheatmeal flour to which malted wheat grains are added. However, many consumers and shops now use the name for other kinds of bread, which usually contain brown flour, with a few bits of whole wheat. Rye flour often finds its way into the loaf. Many people think that the granary is wholemeal. Usually it isn't, although in 1984 Rank Hovis introduced a new loaf called Granary Malted Wholemeal, which does consist of wholemeal flour with added malted wheat grains.

The granary-type bread produced by a good master baker can be a very tasty loaf. But beware – some breads are dyed with caramel. Occasionally you cut them and find swirls of white where the caramel has not been properly mixed!

Hovis and Vit-be are made of flour to which extra germ has been added, so they contain quite large amounts of B vitamins. However they are still not wholemeal, because they do not contain 100 per cent of the whole grain. They lack bran.

Hi-bran and 'bran fortified' breads were created in response to the publicity about dietary fibre. Compared with real wholemeal bread they are sub-standard. They may consist of white flour with quite a lot of bran added. Their fibre value is therefore quite high, but because the germ is usually lacking, nothing like as much of the vitamins and minerals are present as in wholemeal.

Convinced that the British public must have their bread whiter than white, bread factories have brought out the high-fibre white loaf. Maybe this is for those who want to pretend that they care little for nutritional fads and fashions but still want to throw away their laxatives.

This bread contains added vegetable fibre, often from the pea plant, and it most certainly isn't wholemeal. And do not be fooled by clever advertising into thinking that bread made with any old flour will do, just as long as some fibre has been added. Because vegetable fibre is different from cereal fibre. And it does not contain the same vitamins and minerals.

Wholemeal: The Real Thing

Nothing added, nothing taken away, that is the regulation. Wholemeal bread must by law consist of 100 per cent whole wheat, yeast and water. It can contain fat, salt, sugar and only 'natural' baking improvers such as vitamin C. This is the loaf to which we should all be turning. Breakfast, lunch, tea, dinner – wholemeal bread should appear at at least two of your daily meals. But how can you know that it is really wholemeal?

First, you can make your own from 100 per cent wholemeal flour. The cheapest comes from wholefood shops and can often be bought in bulk. Many of these shops sell different kinds of wholemeal flour; ask them which is best.

But not many of us have time to bake bread, and we must rely on our local supermarkets and bakeries. Shop around, be fussy. Ask the assistants if they have wholemeal bread made with 100 per cent of the whole grain. Do not be fobbed off when they say 'we've got wheatmeal', because that is not the same as wholemeal. Nor is Granary (unless it is Granary Malted Wholemeal). Nor Hovis. Nor Brown. Far too many bakery assistants are ignorant about the breads they sell. Ask for 100 per cent wholemeal bread. If the bakery doesn't sell it, go elsewhere. Wholefood shops often sell very good quality wholemeal bread. And so do some supermarkets. Good quality wholemeal bread if solid will keep for a week.

Bread Labels

How can you know what a loaf of bread contains? Wrapped bread, in common with nearly all other packaged foods, must be labelled with its ingredients. But for the purposes of a consumer, what is an ingredient? Well, several additives are put into flour at the milling stage, but all that goes on the bread label is 'flour'. The bakers have been let off the hook: Ministry of Agriculture regulations allow them to pull the wool over consumers' eyes, as well as allowing them to put wool down our throats. If additives go in at the milling stage, then 'flour with additives x, y and z' can be called just 'flour'.

Under new regulations, unwrapped bread has to be labelled at the point of sale; the shop keeper must display a notice giving the list of ingredients. If you are not satisfied, ask to speak to the shop manager, or write to the manufacturer.

Choose your wholemeal bread with care. Since fibre became big business, many new loaves have appeared on the shop shelves. Some have not complied with the regulation that wholemeal means nothing added, nothing taken away. White flour with added bran has been passed off as wholemeal. Real wholemeal bread has a distinctive grainy appearance which is different from the 'added bran' variety.

How Much Bread Should We Eat?

Bread is not very popular. We buy about 2 lb of bread per person per week to eat at home, and perhaps about another 8 oz outside home. The exact amount is difficult to estimate because so much is wasted, or fed to birds and pets.

Some 70 per cent of the bread we eat is white, and most of it is factory-baked. That dreary, tasteless, puffy, glutinous loaf accounts for over 1½ of the 2 lb eaten each week at home. Most of our loaves come from the factories; independent master-bakers make less than a third of our bread. Why we as a nation have come to eat such poor-quality bread, and why good independent master-bakers have all but vanished from the high streets, is a long and sad story. The result is that most large towns have only one or two proper bakers, who need all the support they can get if they are to continue in business. It is the good master-bakers who can supply us with bread made by proper fermentation and without superfluous chemicals. However, few bakeries make this type of bread at the moment.

Make friends with your nearest master-baker. Take an interest in the baking. Find out what sort of flour is used, and how many additives find their way into the mixture. Try new sorts of bread. Visit the Italian and Greek shops; some of their bread is much better quality. Good bread can and should be a pleasure to eat. But we won't get it unless we insist on it.

Wholemeal bread is nutritionally totally superior to white or brown bread. There is no doubt about this. It is richer in fibre and many essential oils, vitamins and minerals found in the whole grain. Ideally all of us should eat it all the time. Six thick slices of wholemeal bread a day would put us all in much better shape.

However, many of us might find it difficult to make a complete change. You can compromise as follows. First, eat bread more often. In less affluent times, British people used to do what many Europeans still do today: eat bread with all their main meals – breakfast, lunch and dinner. But we are unlikely to change our habits unless the quality of our bread improves quite dramatically. A basketful of typical British white sliced bread will hardly make many people drool at the table.

So the recommendation is not just to eat much more bread, but to choose better quality loaves. Better bread does cost more, but over all a healthy diet need not be more expensive. More bread, more potatoes, more fish, more fresh green vegetables and fruit, at the expense of less fatty meat and less processed food.

If you and your family are used to eating only white bread, and do not want to change, at least try some better quality white bread. Visit a local master-baker, or a Greek or Italian shop if there is one in your neighbourhood. Try some of the breads with seeds on top, caraway, poppy and sesame.

When people first eat wholemeal bread they often find it rather heavy, and a few complain of indigestion. Their intestines are not used to the fibre. If it gives you indigestion, introduce it to your diet gradually.

Changing from white to wholemeal bread is rather like giving up sugar or salt. At first you cannot imagine how food could possibly taste right without them. A few months later you wonder how you could possibly have eaten them. Similarly, after eating good-quality bread, a slice of factory-made white pap is of unbelievably bad quality. It has no flavour or texture.

Bread on its own is not fattening. It is the layer of fat that adds the surplus calories. So try to eat less butter and margarine. Good quality bread does not need a layer of fat on

top of it, and can be eaten plain with most main meals. Have
bread with soups and stews. Bread and cheese need no butter:
when did you last see a Frenchman digging into the butter
before cutting a slice of cheese?

Rice, Pasta, Noodles

Some of the finest cooking in the world comes from countries
where rice and pasta are the staple food. Apart from consuming
far too much salt, the Japanese eat very healthily and have the
longest recorded life expectancy of any country in the world.
Plenty of rice, vegetables and fish, only very little fats and
meat. Traditional food in Italy and Greece is also fine. Lots of
starchy bread and pasta, little saturated fats, little meat, lots of
fish, plenty of fruit and vegetables, and olive oil.

We need to look to other cultures to improve our cooking.
There is nothing new or strange about this. Most of the foods
we eat in Britain did not originate here. Potatoes and tomatoes,
for example, came from Latin America. So did most of our
green beans. Rice and pasta are not British inventions any more
than the carrot or cucumber. Our food would seriously lack
variety if it were not for imported agriculture and culinary
skills.

Rice, noodles, pasta and oats are not fattening. The only way
they can become fattening is when loaded with fats and sugars.
If we continue to portray the ideal plate of food as a large lump
of meat, a smallish lump of potato or a pile of rice and another
lump of vegetable, all covered with a fatty sauce, then we have
got it wrong.

A better meal consists of a heap of potatoes, or pasta, or rice,
or noodles, with fish or a little meat, preferably in a tasty sauce
and a lot of vegetables. It is not at all difficult to prepare this
kind of food. Italy, China, southern France, Japan, Greece,
Spain – these countries and many more can show us how to eat
healthy and delicious food.

Many shops now sell brown rice and wholemeal pasta.

Brown rice is actually much easier to cook than white. It takes longer to soften, but the grains do not stick together.

Bread and Cereals – A Summary of the Advice

- Always prefer wholemeal bread. All other bread is inferior. White bread is grossly inferior.

- Eat more bread with main meals.

- Spread the butter and margarine thinly.

- Increase the quantity of cereal foods you eat at the expense of fatty, sugary foods.

- Eat at least six slices of bread a day.

- Brown pastas and rice are best.

- Eat more cereal food of all kinds, especially the whole grain varieties.

CHAPTER 5

Breakfast

CEREALS: WATCH OUT FOR THE SUGARS AND SALT.
MUESLI AND PORRIDGE. COOKED BREAKFASTS:
AVOID THE GREASY SPOON

What does Britain eat for breakfast? When Kelloggs did a survey in the 1970s, they found that only 18 per cent of us ate a cooked breakfast, 40 per cent of us ate breakfast cereals, 25 per cent had bread or toast only, and 17 per cent had nothing at all. This is very different from the 1950s, when half the nation had a cooked breakfast: bacon and eggs were most popular. Less than a quarter of the population ate cereals, and over 90 per cent ate something.

Habits have changed. Over the last thirty years breakfast cereals have become very popular. We eat over twice as much of them as in the 1950s. We eat half as much porridge as we used to. We have no time for bacon and eggs during the week, although we eat them at weekends. We eat less marmalade and less bread, but more of it toasted.

All these changes reflect the way our lives have altered. More women go out to work, have less time to prepare breakfast for their families. We spend less time eating the first meal of the day, and some of us go straight to work without it.

Cereals: Watch Out for Sugars and Salt

Which breakfast cereal do you eat? Is it whole grain? Is it bran enriched, and does this mean it's good for you? Is it as healthy as it claims to be? How much choice do you have among the cardboard boxes in your supermarket?

Breakfast cereal manufacturers have always been rather keen on promoting the healthiness of their products. Goodness, wholesomeness, vigour, strength, vitality, protein, vitamins, minerals – all these qualities are an important part of their advertising message.

Unfortunately, not many breakfast cereals fit the recommendations for a healthier diet, because nearly all of them have added sugars or salt, and occasionally fats. Most are made with processed cereals, not the whole grain.

The manufacturers of Shredded Wheat, Cubs, Mini-Wheats and Puffed Wheat must be congratulated for their continuous production of wholewheat, sugarless, salt-less, fat-less breakfast cereals. Until very recently they had no rivals. All the others were made with varying amounts of sugars and salt, and most were made of processed cereals.

Next time you buy your breakfast cereal, take a look at the list of ingredients. Sugars? Salt? A bowl of Sugar Puffs contains some two or three teaspoons of sugar, and that's before you have reached for the sugar bowl. A bowl of All-Bran has about one teaspoon, cornflakes about one and a half teaspoons. Nearly all of them are sweetened before you start.

Some of them are obviously sweet. The ones that are marketed for young children are usually pretty sickly. But others, such as cornflakes, we tend to think of as unsweetened. We have all become so accustomed to added sweetness that we don't even notice it.

The label doesn't tell you how much has been added.* Nor does it tell you how much salt but, again, few of the

---

*In 1985 Tesco declared the amount of added sugars and salt in their 'own-label' breakfast cereals: a very welcome initiative.

manufacturers are to be congratulated. Some breakfast cereals are rather high in salt: All-Bran, Rice Krispies, cornflakes, Grapenuts, Special K. Would you sprinkle salt on your Shredded Wheat?

Next, the cereal itself. Rice, wheat oats, corn (maize) – these are the basis of most breakfast cereals. Read the labels to find out if it is a hundred per cent whole grain. Many are not.

In response to the craze for fibre, manufacturers have been busy creating new breakfast cereals. Bran flakes, bran buds, bran rings, bran-enriched, bran all over the place. Marketing surveys report that we are also busy buying them. Are they really good for you? A bran-enriched breakfast cereal certainly contains extra fibre, so it is a step in the right direction towards a healthier intestine. If all of us ate a plateful of bran cereal in the morning the country's laxatives bill would fall overnight.

However, just because a cereal has added bran it is not necessarily the best you can buy. We should eat more cereal fibre by choosing wholegrain cereals, not by eating foods to which bran has been indiscriminately added. A reason for this is that bran contains a chemical called phytate which grabs hold of valuable minerals such as zinc and calcium and stops them being absorbed from the intestine into the bloodstream. Wholegrain cereals or wholemeal bread are better foods than bran-enriched breakfast cereals or biscuits. Eaten as the whole mineral-rich grain, the phytate is not a problem.

There is another reason why bran enriched cereals are not as healthy as they sound. A plateful of bran on its own is impossible to eat. It might be just bearable if you swamped it in milk or yoghurt, but munching your way through a bowl of the stuff would not be much of a feast. So how do the bran breakfast cereals come to be edible and dry at the same time? The answer lies in sugars and salt, or even fats, or malt extract. All-Bran and similar products consist of very finely ground bran (whose laxative effect, incidentally, is less powerful than that of coarse bran), sugars about 15 per cent, and salt about 4 per cent. It is the sugars that help to stick the bran together, and make it edible. Bran flakes, bran buds – nearly all the bran breakfast cereals have added sugars and salt. So, despite the added vitamins, and despite the health messages on the packet and advertisements, do not be fooled into thinking this is the ideal breakfast. There are better ways of eating bran.

Muesli

What about muesli? The middle classes have been munching their way through bowlfuls of muesli for several years, and manufacturers have at last realized that not just any old muesli will do. Muesli was invented by the Swiss Doctor M. O. Bircher-Benner and introduced to Britain in the 1930s. The original muesli was rich in fruit. In fact it contained rather more fruit than cereal. It was part of his raw food diet. Over the years the mixture has changed to include more cereal, and since factory production started in Britain it has taken a distinct turn for the worse. Sugars have been introduced, and salt too. Dr Bircher-Benner would turn in his grave. Some mueslis can have as much as 25 per cent added sweeteners, in the form of white sugar, brown sugar, Demerara sugar or honey. The basic message is that all added sweetness is bad news. Muesli containing 10 to 25 per cent sugars is nowhere near as good as muesli without sugars. The list of ingredients gives you a vague idea of what proportion of sugars have been added, because items are listed in order of declining magnitude. In other words, if oats come first on the list, the muesli contains more oats than anything else. If sugar comes before the dried fruit and nuts, then there is likely to be quite a lot of it (unless the manufacturers have been mean with the fruit).

A cunning little trick that is becoming more common is to add sugars as different ingredients: sugar (meaning white sugar), glucose, honey, fructose etc. So the individual amounts look rather small, low down on the list of ingredients. Here is another reason to change the food labelling laws in the interests of consumer freedom. When are we to be allowed to know the sum total of all the different sugars in our food?

Some supermarkets have recently introduced no-salt, no-added sugars muesli which is good news. But if you cannot find a good one, why not make your own? It is very easy. All you need is a bagful of rolled oats, rye, wheat and barley. You can find the mixture in a whole food shop. Then you need chopped dried fruit and nuts – dates, figs, hazelnuts, almonds – anything you like (but not sugar and salt!). Mix the whole lot together and there is your breakfast. You can buy the ingredients in bulk and make enough for a few weeks. The sweetness comes from the dried fruit, and it is even better with fresh fruit on top – apples, bananas, tangerines, pears, peaches. Try it with yoghurt and/or low-fat milk.

Porridge

In 1983, National Oat Week was declared. Porridge used to be a popular breakfast among the poor in Britain, but consumption declined steadily during the first half of the twentieth century, and since the Second World War sales have plummeted even further. This is rather a pity, because oats are a good source of fibre, no doubt the saving grace of the Scottish intestine.

The subject of salt and porridge causes passionate discussion north of the border, and many people are determined that porridge cannot be made any other way. But if you are among those who choose sweet rather than salt porridge, try using less or no salt in cooking. You will get used to it after a few weeks. And try to have a little less sugar as well. Raisins or sultanas in porridge are popular with children and are better than added sugar.

Cooked Breakfasts: Avoid the Greasy Spoon

How big are the slots in your toaster? Could it be that the manufacturers of white sliced plastic-wrapped loaves are in league with the toaster manufacturers? Thick slices just don't fit inside the average modern toaster. As a result, when it comes to toast, the advice to eat thicker slices of better quality bread, particularly wholemeal, often cannot be followed, because so many machines are only designed for the standard slice. If your toaster gives up the ghost, buy one that takes thicker slices.

Eat more bread for breakfast. A couple of slices of wholemeal bread or toast, and not too much butter or marmalade.

The traditional middle class British cooked breakfast was a splendid affair. Kippers, bloaters, fish roes, fish cakes, kidneys, mushrooms and any number of other delicacies were served at this feast. Today we are left with a miserable remnant; a greasy plateful of bacon, eggs and sausage of which some of the worst examples are to be found in cafés frequented by night-shift workers in our cities.

The contents of the average 1980s sausage have already been described; a far cry from the traditional article. Bacon is becoming wetter, but less fatty because of better pig breeding, and some of it is less salty. Eggs from battery chickens are tasteless compared with those of free-range birds.

So if you want a cooked breakfast, what should you choose? Fish cakes (the healthiest and tastiest are probably the ones you make yourself), fish roes, potatoes, mushrooms, tomatoes, lean bacon, the occasional sausage from a reputable butcher, eggs in moderation; all these things are fine. If you fry them, use a good oil. And baked beans or fish fingers are a lot healthier than sausages for children.

Breakfast – A Summary of the Advice

- Choose wholegrain breakfast cereals.
- Avoid cereals with added sugars and salt.
- Eat wholemeal bread.
- Enjoy low-fat cooked breakfasts.

CHAPTER 6

Biscuits and Cakes

CREAM CAKES: NAUGHTY AND NOT NICE.
FLOUR, SUGARS, SALT AND ADDITIVES.
WHAT'S BEST TO BAKE AT HOME.

Since the 1960s we have been eating fewer cakes, scones, teacakes and pastries. This is mainly because fewer of us bother to stop for a meal in mid-afternoon. More women go out to work, and the teatime meal as a formal event has lost popularity, except at weekends.

Home baking is also less popular, although most of all the cakes we eat are still home-made. The instant packet cake so popular in the USA has not really caught on here. Just as well when you look at the ingredients, for many of them consist of little more than refined flour, fats, sugars, colouring, flavouring, the odd bits of dried egg and enough raising agent to blow it up nicely in the oven. Most of the nourishment in the cake comes from the milk and eggs you put into it yourself. As a product, these synthetic cakes are unhealthy, expensive and cannot really be classed as a convenience food, since it takes hardly any less time to make than to start with the basic ingredients; you still have to do the mixing.

This sort of product is a warning to us all of the way in which parts of the food manufacturing industry are progressing, making expensive products out of cheap materials in fancy packets. How would you feel if your own special birthday cake was made like this?

Cream Cakes: Naughty and Not Nice

We may be eating fewer cakes in general, but the popularity of one kind seems to be an ever-upwards swing. 'Naughty but nice', 'Save one for yourself': these are the slogans of the Milk Marketing Board's aggressive advertising campaign on behalf of dairy farmers. So far they have managed to persuade the nation to eat half the cream produced in Britain in the form of cream cakes. In the 1950s hardly anyone ate a cream cake. It was a luxury few could afford, and anyway the traditional British cake just wasn't constructed with cream all over the place. But cream cakes have become big business, and many small bakeries now depend on cakes for a regular income, since they make very little profit from selling bread.

Should you be eating them? Of course you shouldn't! The Milk Marketing Board itself owns up to the fact that they are naughty. Cream, saturated fats, sugars, chocolate, refined flour, salt, artifical flavouring, colouring – these are the main ingredients and none of them are healthy.

Flour, Sugars, Salt, Additives

It has been well and truly instilled in the public mind that cakes and biscuits are fattening, but did you also know that they might be bad for your arteries?

The basic ingredient of cakes and biscuits is flour. As societies become more affluent, instead of eating flour as bread, or dumplings or pasta, they tend to invent more ingenious products using more expensive ingredients. How do you make dry flour palatable and tasty? You can add fat and make pastry.

Or fat and sugar to make biscuits. Or fat, sugar and eggs, to make cakes. The less flour and the more fat, sugar and eggs, the richer the mixture. This is obvious enough to anyone who knows how to cook them, but many people are surprised to learn that cakes and biscuits contain much fat. Men in particular, being generally ignorant still about what goes on in the kitchen, are usually not especially interested in the contents of the digestive biscuit until they learn that their arteries could suffer.

Cakes and biscuits provide over 6 per cent of the saturated fats we eat, according to the Ministry of Agriculture's survey of household food-purchasing habits. This is an underestimate of their total contribution, because so many biscuits, in particular, are eaten outside the home. About a fifth of all biscuits manufactured in 1981 went into the catering trade, and many more are eaten as snacks in offices and factories. What goes into a factory biscuit?

First, the flour. Nearly all manufactured biscuits are made with refined flour. Domestic flour, the sort you buy for cooking, is 72 per cent extraction, which means that the outside 28 per cent of the wheat grain has been removed, leaving the inside 72 per cent which is white flour. Some of the flour the manufacturers use is even more processed. Called 'Patent' flour, it has an extraction rate of only 40 per cent, which means that the outer 60 per cent of the wheat grain has been removed, leaving nothing but white wheat starch. Some products are made of this stuff, but the label on the packet just says 'flour'. So the first problem with a manufactured biscuit is that it is likely to do little for your intestinal health. Highly processed flour bungs you up.

Since the fibre boom in the 1980s, new lines of biscuits have appeared on the supermarket shelves. Added bran, bran biscuits, bran crunch, bran everything. The only way to make dry bran palatable is to load it with sugars, salt and perhaps fats. The stuff has to stick together. Bran biscuits may contain more fibre than their paler counterparts, but most are still packed with sugars and fats. So while a bran or wholemeal biscuit is better than one with white flour, it still doesn't represent health in a packet.

The healthiest way to eat more cereal fibre is to have more wholegrain cereal foods such as wholemeal bread and brown rice. This is because bran taken on its own, without the rest of the grain, can prevent the intestine absorbing essential minerals from food.

The Dreaded 'Seepage'

Second, the fats. Some of the biscuit manufacturers take advantage of the fact that they are not required to tell you exactly which fats they use. The cheap processed fats they buy may be a mixture of several kinds. The important thing from their point of view is that the consistency is uniform, so that the final product looks, feels and tastes the same. The filling must not leak out of a wafer biscuit sitting on the shop shelf at a warmish room temperature. The chocolate coating must not melt and ruin the design imprinted on it. The biscuits must not stick together. All this means that the biscuit filling or topping must be made with a hard fat mixture. In other words, saturated. Filled biscuits are made almost exclusively with palm or coconut oil, both highly saturated in the natural state and further saturated, or hardened, when they are turned into the filling. Furthermore, it is not only the fats used in the filling or the topping that are saturated. Most biscuit shortening is also highly saturated, and the fats can account for one third of the weight of the biscuit.

Look at the Label

What does the label tell you? Biscuit and cake manufacturers are obliged to tell you the ingredients of all wrapped products with a list in descending order of weight. They do not have to specify the extraction rate of the flour, nor the additives put into flour at the milling stage, nor the quantities of fats and sugars, nor the degree of saturation of the fats. Biscuit fat is generally labelled 'vegetable oil or fat', or 'hydrogenated vegetable oil' (that is, saturated). Occasionally butter is specified, or a particular type of vegetable oil. You can assume that most biscuits contain a good deal of saturated fats. The only ones that don't will most likely be presented as health foods. If it says that the oil is soya, sunflower or corn, then it is low in saturated fats.

Third, the sugars. All of us know that sweet biscuits contain sugars, but how about plain or cheese biscuits, cream crackers, water biscuits? Next time you think of buying one of these varieties, take a look at the label. It is astonishing how many 'savoury' foods contain added sugars in the form of sucrose, or maltose, dextrose, glucose or syrups, and how our palates have become so accustomed to the stuff that we don't even detect its presence.

More than half the weight of some sweet biscuits is sugars, which provide no nourishment whatsoever except for energy or calories. Filled and chocolate biscuits are the chief culprits. But some apparently less sweet varieties are still very sugary – semi-sweet biscuits, 22 per cent; digestive, 16 per cent sugar. Processed flour stuck together with fats and sugars: a gluey mess designed to coat teeth with the perfect food for bacteria. It's not just sweets that cause holes in teeth.

Fourth, what next? Apart from flour, fats and sugars, nearly all biscuits contain salt, flavouring and colouring, and a plethora of antioxidants, preservatives, improvers, stabilizers etc.

The news is bad. If you want to care for your health, don't eat so many. Give children a sandwich or a piece of fruit instead of a biscuit; or some malt bread, or a currant bun. True, biscuits are convenient, just the right size and shape for a toddler to hold on to, and sweet enough. But do you really want to bring your child up on food lacking healthy nourishment?

All these comments about manufactured biscuits apply equally well to cakes. Main ingredients: flour, sugars, saturated fats, colouring, flavouring, improvers, raising agents and so on.

Eggs? Home-made cakes usually have a few, but a lot of factory-produced lines are eggless. This might be good news for our blood cholesterol, but might also surprise those who regard eggs as a compulsory cake ingredient. Most cakes are high in sugars; anything from a third to over a half of the weight of a cake can be sugars. Worst culprits? Fancy iced cakes. Icing is pure sugar, give or take a bit of colouring or artificial flavour.

Cake fats are inclined to be saturated, like that of factory biscuits, but you have no way of knowing because the label does not tell you. And again, the flour is highly processed.

What's Best to Bake at Home

Home-made cakes and biscuits are certainly likely to taste better than the average factory-made article, but nevertheless, usually they are not healthy food and are best kept for special occasions. Lard, butter and many margarines are highly saturated fats. Try using margarines labelled 'high in polyunsaturates' or even an oil. You will have to experiment a little with different kinds of fats, but it is possible to make cakes with oil instead of hard fats. Select recipes low in sugars. Better still, make fruit cakes and avoid sugars altogether, relying instead on dry sultanas, currants and dates for sweetness.

Scones, fruit bread, currant buns, malt loaves and teacakes are usually lower in fats and sugars than most cakes and biscuits. They are a healthier choice.

It is worthwhile reflecting that our current passion for sugar is a modern habit. Those who refuse to eat the stuff and avoid it at all cost find most cakes and biscuits unbearably sweet and sickly. Avoiding sugary foods is not easy if you are used to eating 2 lb of sugars every week, the national average. It takes time to adapt. If you eat cakes or biscuits every day, try reducing to alternate days to start with. Have fresh fruit or a sandwich instead.

Biscuits and Cakes – A Summary of the Advice

- Choose less sweet varieties – teacakes, scones, malt loaves, currant buns, fruit and nut cakes.

- Eat cakes and biscuits less often.

- Have fresh fruit or a sandwich instead.

CHAPTER 7

Salt

HOW BIG ARE THE HOLES IN YOUR POT?
CEREALS: LOOK AT THE LABEL. MEAT AND SALTY VEG.
SODIUM FIZZ. WHAT ABOUT CRAMPS?

Does added salt prevent you getting cramp? If you stopped eating salt tomorrow, would you collapse in a faint? On a hot day would you become dizzy and ill without it?

The fact is that none of these things is likely to happen if we all stopped adding salt to our food. The amount of salt the body needs is minute, much less than we eat every day. On average, we eat over ten to twenty times more salt than our bodies require.

The evidence about salt and blood pressure is still not clear. But one thing is clear, and that is that anyone who wants to eat less salt finds it very difficult to buy low-salt processed foods. For until recently, almost every tinned and packaged food on the supermarket shelf has had added salt in it. Have you ever seen tinned spaghetti, or cornflakes, or sausages, without added salt? Why are we not offered a choice? If most processed foods were low in salt, those who like salt could simply add it themselves.

Throw away the salt pot today, and religiously avoid every

food with added salt. If you do this you will find your food tasteless, even uneatable. But if you persevere for a few weeks, you will find your craving for salt surprisingly reduced. People who give up salt are often astonished at how quickly their taste buds adapt. Once you are used to salt-less foods, their natural flavour actually becomes more pronounced. Instead of bringing out the flavour, you find that salt has been covering it up for years. Years and years of lost flavour, and nobody ever told you!

Your body requires less than 1 gram of salt per day. Your total requirement is less than one tenth of the amount we usually eat.

We have no physiological need for extra salt in our food because cereals, vegetables, fruit, meat and milk all contain it in small amounts. Milk actually contains rather a lot, because calves need it. Even milk-less diets contain plenty of salt for human survival and health. Added salt is completely unnecessary in normal conditions.

In nature, all types of food—cereal, vegetable, fruit, meat—contain sparing amounts of sodium, and are rich in potassium. Our problem is not only that we consume far too much sodium, but also that, because so much of our food is highly processed, we consume relatively small amounts of potassium. As a result the natural balance between potassium and sodium in our food and in our bodies is thrown right out. Now that we don't need to preserve food with salt, you can enjoy potassium-rich whole food, fresh or frozen, and in this respect enjoy better health than your grandparents.

How Big are the Holes in Your Pot?

Salt used to be very expensive. Indeed, it was so valuable that it used to be used as currency. (The word 'salary' derives from it.) To sit below the salt at table was a sign of poverty and low social worth. Nowadays it is smart to sit below the salt. You might live longer.

You could chuck your salt-pot away, or lock it up as an interesting by-gone. Try to reduce the amount your children eat. Better still is not to start them off on the habit of sprinkling salt on their food. ·

Do you pour salt on to your food before you have tasted it? A lot of people do. You can see them in restaurants, reaching for the pot to ruin the flavour of the food they haven't even tasted.

How big are the holes in your salt pot? Big holes let out more salt. By sneakily changing the size of the holes in salt pots in restaurants, researchers have discovered that they can change the amount of salt people eat, without their knowing! It seems that a lot of the salt we eat is because of habit rather than taste.

Boiled in Brine?

Adding salt when you cook vegetables does not improve their quality. It does not make them greener, or healthier. When you cook vegetables, do you first fill the saucepan with water, then add a couple of teaspoons of salt, then put the vegetables in to float?

Cooked vegetables have most flavour when cooked in the absolute minimum of boiling water, without salt. Steamed vegetables are even better. Spinach is best cooked with no water at all; it makes its own juice and does not burn provided you start cooking it gently. Potatoes, too, taste better cooked without salt once you are used to them. The world's great chefs have now started to revise their ideas about salt, for gastronomic rather than health reasons. It is now quite common to find them cooking vegetables without it, relying instead on natural flavours.

What about meat, fish and eggs? To many people, the idea of cooking fish and eggs without salt is insane. Surely they would be totally devoid of flavour? Yet the art of cooking without salt is not simply to avoid the salt pot, but to look for alternative flavours. Herbs, spices and lemon juice should be in every kitchen.

If you are usually heavy-handed with salt, make a conscious effort to use less. Do it gradually, and your family probably won't even notice.

Table and cooking salt are under our own control. Salt in manufactured foods is not. There are no regulations about the amount of salt allowed in processed foods, and nothing on food labels to say how much the manufacturer has added. Why is this information kept from us?

Take a look at the labels of tinned, bottled and packet foods. You'll be lucky to find more than half a dozen in a large supermarket without added salt, although one or two of the leading chains now offer a few salt-less items. Our tastebuds are delivered a constant dose of salt, without our even noticing.

Cereals: Look at the Label

All-Bran is one of the worst offenders. Would you believe that it is about 4 per cent salt? Cornflakes and Rice Krispies are only marginally better at about 3 per cent. Next come Bran Flakes, Special K, Grapenuts, Weetabix and many, many more. Our breakfast can be a salty affair.

By contrast, Shredded Wheat, Puffed Wheat and some mueslis contain none, so clearly it is possible to create popular cereals without salt.

Why do the manufacturers add it? First, they think we want it. Second, some of their products so lack alternative flavour that without salt few of us would get interested. Some of the bran cereals are a good example. The only way to turn bran into a tempting meal is to stick it together with sugars and salt.

Choose your breakfast cereal after reading the label. Look for the whole grain varieties without salt. Look for unsalted, unsweetened muesli; or you could make your own instead.

Peanuts, crisps and other snacks can be extremely salty.

Choose unsalted peanuts instead. Eat crisps less often. They are not a regular healthy snack for children because they are so salty. If you want to eat less, try fresh fruit or a sandwich instead. Give children raisins and unsalted nuts. Some manufacturers have started packaging them in little boxes popular with tiny fingers.

Meat and Salty Veg

Until now, nearly all canned vegetables have had sugars and salt added, with the exception of some tomatoes. Some manufacturers have now decided that it is time to offer the British public a choice of unsalted vegetables. So, if you read the labels, you might find you're in luck. If you cannot find vegetables without salt, buy frozen instead. Better still, buy them fresh. Canned baked beans, butter beans and kidney beans are all salted (unless they say 'no added salt' on the label).

Tinned and processed meat always contains added salt. In sausages, hams and similar products, the salt is partly used as a preservative. Before the days of refrigeration, drying and salting meat (and vegetables) was the only way to keep them through the winter. Today we have fridges and freezers. So do shops. There is no need to tip salt into all these meat products, because they are transported in cold lorries and sold from a chilled shelf, or from the freezer.

Bacon, black puddings and salamis are the most salty, at about 3 to 6 per cent of their total weight. Next come hams, corned beef, haggis, tongue, faggots, chopped ham and Spam, at about 2 to 3 per cent salt.

By contrast, fresh meat contains very little salt. To reduce your intake, eat fewer sausages and pies. Most of these things are also very fatty, so you would be better off eating less of them anyway.

Bacon and ham are much less salty (and fatty) than they used to be. One or two supermarkets are leading the way in producing less salty bacon, but they still do not tell you how much has been added. Buy unsmoked rather than smoked.

Dried and tinned soups are particularly salty. If you always eat them, you probably won't notice it. Years of consumption of 57 salted varieties have worn a hole in your tastebuds. A healthier choice is more home-made soups instead. They do not take long to cook, and are easily made with a blender.

There's more salt in nearly all pickles and sauces. Some sweet pickles are 5 per cent salt, tomato ketchup 3 per cent, piccalilli 3 per cent, and salad cream 2 per cent. Pickles could be made without salt; the vinegar will do the preserving. Chutney made with vinegar but without salt keeps perfectly well. Bought salad cream can be replaced with home-made French dressing. All you need is a good-quality oil and a little vinegar or lemon juice, and maybe some herbs.

Manufactured sauces often contain sugar as well as salt, so less is best. Try not to bring children up on food swamped with tomato sauce.

Sodium Fizz

Do soft drinks contain salt? Ordinary salt is sodium chloride. But there are other sources of sodium in our food (the sodium is probably the harmful part). Many fizzy canned and bottled drinks contain sodium (as sodium citrate). It adds flavour. And soda water is full of sodium. Read the labels to find out how many sodium chemicals these drinks contain. Don't forget that unless they say they are made with real fruit juice (and even then it may only be a fairly minute amount), most soft drinks consist entirely of water, sugars, colouring, flavouring and fizz. They are rotten value for money.

Buy unsalted or 'slightly salted' butter. Some health food shops sell unsalted margarine, high in polyunsaturates.

All bread is salted. One reason is because salt is cheaper than wheat. You have no control over the quantity used in manufacture, and furthermore the label does not tell you how much has been used.

Is salt necessary in baking? Many cooks are convinced that it improves baking quality, but there is no evidence that they are correct. Pastry, bread, cakes and biscuits can all be made successfully without it.

Many additives contain sodium, for example monosodium glutamate, sodium polyphosphate, sodium citrate, sodium bicarbonate – there are many more.

Maggi bouillon cubes on sale in Greece in summer 1984 were found to contain over 40 per cent salt, and 12 per cent monosodium glutamate; the label said so in Greek and English!

What About Cramps?

Do you need extra salt in hot weather? In 1983, we had a hot summer, and it was announced on the news that people should take extra salt to avoid dizziness. Was the advice correct?

Once the conventional advice for anyone travelling to the tropics was that salt tablets were essential for survival. However, we now know that our bodies adapt to hot temperatures.

After a week or two in a hot environment, the amount of salt sweat contains is much reduced. The body acclimatizes so as to conserve essential salts. The rapid changes of temperature that a plane journey from London to Africa produces can upset the salt balance, and initially salt loss in sweat will be high. It is now understood that the armed forces need time to adapt before engaging in strenuous activities in hot places. Salt tablets are not necessary as a rule.

Added salt in food is also unnecessary in Britain, even in summer. Enough salt occurs naturally in food to prevent ill effects. And the added salt in bread, cheese, bacon and ham which most of us eat means that we all eat well in excess of our salt requirements.

The only problems are likely to be with people whose body

temperature alternates rapidly between very hot and cold. Miners have been advised to take extra salt for this reason.

Many middle-aged people develop cramp in their limbs, especially their legs, which can be extremely painful. The cause is generally unknown, but it is extremely unlikely to be lack of salt in the diet. Extra salt does not usually stop these cramps.

Salt Substitutes

In response to warnings about the dangers of salt in food, some salt substitutes have appeared in chemist shops and supermarkets. Most are a mixture of sodium chloride and potassium chloride. A few are potassium chloride alone. They are expensive. Potassium chloride does have a salty flavour, but it also has a bitter after-taste. These substitutes are not harmful, since our diet is rather low in potassium. But extra potassium is much better derived from whole cereal grains, fruits and vegetables than from a pot of potassium chloride.

An interesting new salt substitute has been developed in the USA. It is derived from strains of food yeasts, and is low in potassium and sodium, while still having a salty flavour. Its flavour is very convincing. However, it is much more expensive than ordinary salt and potassium chloride.

Try using less salt in general, and cultivate a taste for unsalted food, rather than relying on a substitute.

In general, you must read the food labels in order to avoid salt in manufactured foods. They do not tell you how much salt has been added, nor if the salt content of the food is high, medium or low. If manufacturers developed a code, it would help us all to distinguish between the most and least salty foods. And it would give us all greater choice.

Salt – A Summary of the Advice

• Read food labels; avoid salty food.

- Eat more fresh foods.
- Use less salt in cooking.
- Use more herbs, spices, lemon juice instead.
- Use less salt at the table.
- Aim to give up the salt pot altogether.
- Never give salt to babies and toddlers.

CHAPTER 8

Sugars

SUGARS PROVIDE EMPTY CALORIES.
PACKETS OF SUGAR VERSUS SUGAR IN PACKETS.
A NEW GAME: HUNT THE SUGARS IN YOUR FOOD.

Every year, 100 lb of sugar for every man, woman and child in the country disappear down the collective British gullet. We have been told and told that the stuff is bad for us. So why do we still eat it?

Many people believe that sugar is essential for health and energy. Word has got about that without added sugar in our food we would all faint and keel over. This belief has arisen because sugars for many years have been classified as an 'energy' food. True, they do provide energy, or calories. But that does not mean that we will lack vital energy without them, for our bodies derive energy from all the foods we eat – meat, eggs, milk, cheese, bread, potatoes, oranges. All of them provide energy.

What is sugar anyway? Glucose, sucrose, fructose, fructose syrup B.P., dextrose, maltose, brown sugar, white sugar, treacle, demerara sugars, cane sugar, golden syrup, molasses, honey – are they all as different as they sound, and are some of them better for you than others? Are any of them beneficial?

Sugar and the British Diet – Have We Always Eaten It?

Sugar cane was first cultivated in India in the third century BC. It spread slowly through China, Arabia, the Mediterranean, Africa and then the Americas. The sugar refined from it could be bought for a price, but only by the very wealthy. In fact it was so expensive that the lucky owners used to lock it up in little boxes. Its price was rather like that of caviar today. It was only about 200 years ago that the price fell so much that it was eaten in any quantity.

During the eighteenth century, slavery meant that the Caribbean sugar-cane plantations expanded, prices fell, and demand grew. But sugar was still an expensive luxury for the mass of the British population, even though the rich regularly ate it by now. They began to create sweet puddings. The poor started to put sugar in their tea. Cheaper than butter, treacle oozed its way on to the labourer's bread.

Being a luxury, sugar was taxed. But in 1874 the duty was lifted, and the price fell considerably. This was the point of departure; from now on sugar was no longer regarded as a luxury but as a regular, normal part of everyday food. By the beginning of the twentieth century, jam was being mass-produced. Cakes and biscuits could be bought for a price, but were still a luxury for the poor. Out of all the countries in the world, Britain became the most addicted to sweet food. Throughout the twentieth century, despite disruptions to supplies and rationing during two world wars, consumption of sugar was steadily increased. We now eat around 2 lb per head per week.

The history of sugar consumption tells us one thing quite clearly. For all but a blink of an eye in the history of life on this planet, refined sugars have been an unknown commodity. There was just one exception – honey – and even that was a luxury. Refined sugars did not exist, except by courtesy of the bees. Our ancestors' food consisted of large quantities of fruit, vegetables and cereals, together with some animal foods. All the sugars in their diet came together with the rest of the plant, and for millions of years our ancestors lived without it being artificially extracted and refined.

Until recently, there were still a few societies which had escaped the inexorable spread of stickiness. But sugar production and trading is an international business with immense profitability. Sugar is cheap to produce, it is easily transported, does not go bad, can be stock-piled indefinitely waiting for prices to improve, can be tipped into processed foods with astonishing ease, and can be sold to the poor the world over. Where soft drinks and sweets were once unheard of, today they are commonplace. Africa, India, Asia and Latin America now wallow in sweetness, and their health is beginning to suffer. Even the Chinese, whose consumption of sugars used until recently to be infinitesimal by world standards, now get through about 11 lb per person per year. Sweet and sour pork, ridiculed by the Chinese restaurateurs of Europe and America, may yet become the favourite dish in Peking. The world sugar trade has an ambition, and that is to see every country in the world guzzling its way through an average of 2 lb of sugar per person per week. In Britain they have succeeded.

What are Sugars

Plants make sugars and store them in their stems and roots. Carrots, swedes, turnips, sugar beet, beetroot, sugar cane – all these plants, and many more, make stores of sugars and, left to their own devices, would use them as energy for making flowers and seeds, and for next year's spring growth.

How is the sugar extracted? Seven pounds of sugar cane makes one pound of sugar; one huge sugar beet makes a teaspoon of sugar. The sugar has to be separated from the fibrous plant material. The juice is squeezed out, concentrated into syrup or crystals, cleaned, purified, bleached, crystallized, turned into lumps, ground into caster and icing sugar, put into packets. 'White, refined sugar is one of the purest foods known to man, it is 99.9 per cent pure', the Sugar Bureau (formerly called the British Sugar Bureau) proudly proclaimed in their 1983 booklet 'Sweet Reason', sent free to health professionals throughout the country to extol the virtues and health benefits of sugar in food. Pure and sweet it certainly is, but the amount of reason in this book is a matter of debate. The Sugar Bureau is a Central London-based organization which, like the Butter Information Council, or the Flora Information Service, is an organization set up specifically to promote the consumption of a particular product. Its chief purpose is to maintain and increase its share of the market. To make sure we all continue to munch our way through fields full of sugar beet and sugar cane for the greater glory of the beet-producers and the plantation owners. Sugar is big business.

Here are the different kinds of cane and beet sugars that find their way into our food, in approximate order of refinement.

The Syrups

Molasses

Sugar-cane molasses is quite expensive. It is thick and black and has a strong, almost bitter, flavour. It is the residue from the first crystallization process. The cane is squeezed, the juice is dried, the crystals removed and what is left is molasses. Molasses can also be made from sugar beet, but it is used mainly for animal feed. Molasses is about 30 per cent water and 5 per cent minerals. All the rest is sugar.

Black Treacle

This comes next in the league of refinement. It is a thinner version of molasses, slightly more diluted and a little less bitter. It is about 30 per cent water and 3 per cent minerals, and all the rest is sugar.

Golden Syrup
This is made of refined sugar cane or beet sugar. It is about 20 per cent water and contains caramel colouring (made from refined sugars) or a little molasses. It contains less than 1 per cent of minerals.

The Sugars

Brown Sugars
These are either raw, made from crystallized cane juice with a strong flavour and brown colour, or manufactured, made from white sugar to which a little molasses, or treacle, or caramel colouring has been added for flavour and colour. Brown sugars are either soft and brown, or more gritty and paler yellow (demerara sugars).

i *Raw soft brown sugars*
   If the label says 'raw cane sugar', and states the country of origin (for example Barbados), and if the sugar is called Barbados, or Molasses sugar, or Muscovado sugar, then it is raw, soft brown cane sugar. This sugar has a rich smell and strong taste.

ii *'Manufactured' soft brown sugars*
    These are all called 'soft' but not raw. They may have a list of ingredients (sugar, caramel, molasses) and they do not give a country of origin. Basically, they are dyed white sugar.

iii *Raw cane demerara sugars*
     This sugar is called demerara, raw cane sugar, and the label shows the country of origin. Its smell and taste are stronger than its 'manufactured' counterpart.

iv *'Manufactured' demerara sugars*
    What distinguishes this from its 'raw' demerara neighbour is the fact that the label gives no country of origin. It is

called 'demerara (sugar and cane molasses)' or 'demerara (cane sugar and cane molasses)'. These are dyed white sugars.

White Sugars

White sugars (sucrose) are marketed in several different forms, all of them only too familiar.

Preserving sugars: bigger crystals than granulated sugar.
Granulated sugars: ordinary, white, packet sugar.
Caster and icing sugars: ground-up white sugar.
Coffee crystals: large crystals, sometimes dyed brown with caramel.
Sugar cubes: white sugar stuck together to make lumps.

The types of sugars listed above are all derived from sugar cane and sugar beet. As such, their main, and usually their only, ingredient is sucrose. Sucrose chemically is part made of fructose, part glucose.

Other Forms of Sugar

But sucrose is not the only sugar to find its way into our food. An increasing number of other types of sugars are being tipped into cauldrons in food factories. Glucose, fructose, lactose, maltose, dextrose, invert sugar. What are these things? Are they very different from ordinary white sugar (sucrose)? Are they healthy, are they villains, or is our metabolism indifferent to their presence?

First, a look at what they are.

Glucose

Glucose is the sugar found in grape juice, and is the stuff the wine producers rely on to turn into alcohol during fermentation. It occurs naturally in all fruit and vegetable juices. We make it in our own bodies.

The food industry is using much more glucose than it used

to. In 1982, each of us ate on average more than 16 lb glucose in processed foods. Glucose is a bit less sweet than sucrose.

Dextrose
Dextrose is another name for pure glucose.

Fructose
Fructose (also known as laevulose) is the sweetest known naturally occurring sugar, twice as sweet as sucrose. Honey contains fructose, as do some fruits and vegetables.

In the USA a great deal of money is now being made out of the production, and sale to the food manufacturing industries, of high fructose corn syrup. Maize varieties which produce large amounts of fructose sugar have been produced. This is of course a major threat to the sugar cane and sugar beet producers around the world, because fructose is twice as sweet as ordinary white sugar; therefore the manufacturers only need half the quantity.

The reaction of the UK and the EEC to high fructose corn syrup was to slap an import quota on to it at the first opportunity in order to protect EEC sugar beet production. This was bad luck for those who thought they might make a tidy little sum from importing it into the UK.

In terms of our health, fructose is an improvement on the less sweet sugar cane and sugar beet varieties (because the same sweetness comes in half the quantity). But better still would be none at all.

Lactose
Lactose is milk sugar. All milks contain it, including human and cows'. It is one sixth as sweet as sucrose.

Maltose
Malt extract contains maltose, which is one of the products of beer making and comes from barley. It is a third as sweet as sucrose.

Invert sugar
Invert sugar is popular with confectionery manufacturers because it does not crystallize. It contains glucose and fructose, and is made by treating sucrose with acids. Invert sugar is a little less sweet than sucrose.

Glucose syrup
Glucose syrup is made from corn (maize) starch. It is a bit less sweet than glucose, and is increasingly being used in food manufacture.

Maple Syrup
This comes from the North American maple tree. It is largely sucrose and water.

Honey
Honey contains glucose and fructose. It is 20 to 25 per cent water. The flavour of honey comes from the aroma of flowers. These fragrant chemicals account for only a minute fraction of a jar of honey. The sweetness of honey varies a good deal, depending on the water content and the type of flowers visited by the bees.

Sorbitol
Sorbitol is sugar alcohol. It is half as sweet as sucrose, and is used in some slimming and diabetic products. Eaten in large amounts, it can cause diarrhoea.

The Nutritional Value of Sugars

So much for the different types of sugars in our food. What about their nutritional value?

All sugars are carbohydrates, but not all carbohydrates are sugars as we think of them. This is important, because we have all been taught that carbohydrates are evil, fattening, useless things, to be avoided at all cost. But the truth is that there are carbohydrates and carbohydrates, and they are by no means all the same.

Starches, dietary fibre and sugars – all of them are carbohydrates.

One of the most crucial messages of this book is to explain that starch and sugar are not the same thing. Starches naturally occurring together with dietary fibre equals healthy wholegrain cereals, potatoes, rice, pasta, noodles. Sugars, naturally occurring together with dietary fibre, equals healthy fruit and vegetables. But processed ('refined') sugars of all types by themselves equal empty energy, providing no nourishment but only calories.

Sugars Provide Empty Calories

The different sugars described on pages 213–217 have one thing in common. They are all highly concentrated forms of simple sugars. Occurring in small quantities in plants, these sugars have been concentrated to make sugar as we know it. (Remember the 7 lb sugar cane that make 1 lb sugar?) Nutritional analysis of all these sugars reveals that, with the exception of molasses, black treacle and raw sugars, energy or calories is all they provide, give or take the odd molecule of calcium and magnesium. White sugars, manufactured brown sugars, fructose, glucose – all of them provide absolutely nothing of value whatever apart from calories. No vitamins. No minerals. No fibre. No protein. No starches. *Nothing but calories.* Even black treacle and molasses provide so few minerals in comparison with the amount of sucrose that they are not worth eating. For this reason all these sugars are called EMPTY CALORIES, and for this reason they have no place in a healthy diet. For every wretched spoonful of sugars we eat, we could be eating many, many more spoonfuls of nutritious food providing vitamins, minerals, fibre, proteins and starch. Sugars added to our food literally displace healthy nutrients from our diet.

This fact is difficult to understand, because three spoonfuls of sugar dissolved in a cup of tea do not seem to displace anything. The sugar has dissolved, the tea is still there, so what has been displaced? Sugars affect appetite. Hunger can be satisfied with a packet of boiled sweets, but what nutritional value have they provided other than calories? None. Furthermore, sugars can affect appetite in other directions. The more sugars you eat, the more you want, the more empty calories you consume at the expense of nutritious foods.

We consume on average around 2 lb of sugars per head per week – about 3,400 calories, more than enough for a day's existence for a woman or child, and more than enough for all but the big or active. Processed sugars supply, on average, one in every five calories we eat.

The NACNE report said we should halve our present intake of sugars. A certain amount of fudging was involved in setting the figure at half of our present consumption, for no decent dietitian or nutritionist nowadays would include any refined sugars at all in a perfect, healthy diet. Most dentists actively concerned with preventing dental decay recommend that refined sugars should vanish from our diet.

How can you reduce the sugars you consume? Where are sugars to be found in our food?

Packets of Sugar Versus Sugar in Packets

Between 1955 and 1980, the amount of packet sugar bought by households fell by 37 per cent: a most encouraging sign.

Have we been buying less packet sugar because we are conscious of its harmful effects? The rising sales of artificial sweeteners for tea and coffee certainly suggest that this is so.

We also use less sugar because we do less home baking. Housewives make fewer puddings, jams, biscuits and cakes and go out to work instead. 'Tea' as a meal has been on the decline for several years.

We also seem to be developing a preference for savoury rather than sweet food. Fewer packets of sugar, more cheese, more cheese and savoury biscuits; fewer cakes, less jam, less marmalade, more savoury snacks – this is the trend shown by Ministry of Agriculture analyses of the British shopping basket over the last few years. It certainly looks as if we are going right off the sweet stuff.

But hold on a minute. When did you last look at the list of contents of a tin of tomato soup, or baked beans, or peas, or muesli, or Spam, or pickled cucumbers, or cheese biscuits, fruit yoghurt, savoury rice, tomato sauce, barbecue relish, garlic sausage, smoked ham, tinned ravioli, beefburgers, Cumberland pie, Worcester sauce, pork sausages, macaroni cheese, cornflakes, sweetcorn, red kidney beans? There are sugars in all that lot! Have we gone mad? Our meals have been turned on their heads. When did you last sprinkle sugar on your roast beef and Yorkshire pudding, or on to the cabbage? Crazy you might think, but that is exactly what the food industry gets up to on our behalf. For as fast as we have been studiously avoiding the stuff in our tea and coffee and trying to eat fewer over-sweetened cakes because we know they are bad for us, the food manufacturers have been shovelling it right back into our food before it hits the supermarket trolley. While our household purchases of packet sugar have declined by a third since the 1950s, the total amount of all refined sugars we eat remains at a stubborn 2 lb per head per week. It is quite true that the total quantity of ordinary white sugar (sucrose, from sugar cane and sugar beet) has declined. But as fast as it has declined, the consumption of other sugars, particularly glucose, has gone up. And all except a tiny amount of these are eaten in manufactured foods, both sweet and savoury.

To claim that as a nation we now prefer savoury food is nonsense. We may buy more packets of savoury biscuits, but it's a funny kind of savoury that contains added sugars.

What is the food industry doing? Why is it so keen to make

us eat this harmful substance? The answer is that EEC and government subsidies between them make sugar production an extremely profitable business. With so much economic support, the price is cheap. It costs less than nutritious food. And if it is cheap, in it goes. Never mind if the food is sweet or savoury; the proportion in sweetened foods is so large that all of us are used to eating sugar in nearly all our processed foods.

There is another reason why the food industry likes to put sugar into everything. It is not only a cheap bulking agent, it also makes sauces thick, it sticks things together, and it provides something the food industry loves to talk about: 'mouth feel'. Mouth feel is apparently what you get when you drink a canful of Coca-Cola. Seven teaspoons of sugar per can give a syrupy feel to the liquid that artificial sweeteners cannot match. This is 'positive mouth feel'. But to those who avoid sugar like the plague, mouth feel is sickly, sweet, gooey. Only when you have religiously avoided sugar for some months do you appreciate the over-sweetness of many everyday foods.

Where is the sugar in your food? Most of us think we are eating less than we used to. Ask anyone how much sugar they eat, and you will often get the reply 'oh, I've cut down a lot: I don't have it at all in tea or coffee any more.' Then you say 'What about cakes and biscuits?' and find they are on the way out too. Well, if all of us are, on average, maintaining national consumption of all sugars at 2 lb per head per week, then someone is eating it. Who, and where?

The answer is to be found on labels of soft drinks, and sweet and savoury foods. But it is not an instantly understandable message. For when the manufacturer is obliged to list the ingredients (in order of content) on the packet, 'sugar' applies only to the ordinary white stuff. All other sugars and modified sugars are called by different names and here they are:

Sucrose
Glucose, glucose syrup

Dextrose, dextrose syrup
Fructose, fructose syrup
Maltose, maltose syrup
Invert sugar
Caramel
Sorbitol

Not to mention 'brown', 'pure' and 'raw' sugar. So when you examine the list of contents of a biscuit, you may find the word 'sugar' quite a long way down the list. You may even think the variety of biscuits is quite healthy. But elsewhere in the list, you are increasingly likely to find a sprinkling of all sorts of other sugars. The problem for consumers is that manufacturers are not obliged to add up the *total content* of added sugars. If sugars were listed as such in the list of ingredients, many food labels would begin with the words 'total added sugars', rather than 'flour'. The other problem is that ingredients are often given for different parts of the food separately, so swiss roll has one list of ingredients for the cake mixture, and another one for the filling. It is of course absolutely right that as long as the industry uses all these substances, the public should be informed about their presence. But with increasingly complex concoctions going into what many of us regard as everyday foods, when is the government going to develop labelling regulations that really do benefit the consumer? And of course the much bigger question is: when is the government going to review the whole system of manufacture that encourages the production of 'foods' which consist of nothing more than refined flours, refined sugars, processed fats, colourings, flavourings and preservatives, not to mention the odd pesticide residue?

A New Game: Hunt the Sugars in Your Food

There is a further problem with sugars, which again makes it well nigh impossible for us to know exactly how much we are eating. Small amounts of added sugars do not always have to be declared in the ingredient list. So 'fruit juice' can contain up to 15 grams per litre (that's half an ounce) before it has to be labelled as 'sweetened'. Crystallized fruit of course contains sugar, but if the amount of fruit used does not exceed 10 per cent by weight of the food, the sugar in it need not be declared. Similarly, chocolate, jam, and a host of other things, if used as an ingredient in less than a specified quantity, do not have to be declared with a full list of their ingredients. The labelling laws are very complicated indeed. It would take most of us many months to understand.

Breakfast Cereals

Most breakfast cereals contain added sugars. Sugar Puffs, Sugar Smacks, Coco-Pops, Rice Krispies, All-Bran, Alpen, the list is endless. Shredded Wheat, Cubs, Mini-Wheats, Puffed Wheat are free of sugar, together with some mueslis that have recently appeared on the market.

Read the label. Watch out for 'sugar' but also 'syrup' and any ingredient ending in '-ose'. Honey, brown sugar, raw sugar – it's all basically the same stuff, often described as 'energy-giving' to start your day with a bang.

Do you put sugar on to an already sweetened cereal? If so, why? Most of us use sugar out of habit. We have become accustomed to the taste. Try eating half as much. You will be surprised how soon you get used to it. Try unsweetened mueslis. Rely on fresh and dried fruit for sweetness instead.

Tea and Coffee

The same argument applies. Sugar is habit-forming, addictive. The more you eat it the more you want it. Try taking half as much sugar in your drinks; even a third less is a good start. Make a conscious effort to kick the habit. Some people find it best to give it all up in one go, others do it more slowly. If you complain that being asked to eat less sugar is being asked to forgo a major pleasure in life, consider that other people's habits and addictions are seen for what they really are. They seldom look like pure pleasure. The hardened sugar eater is probably just as habituated to the stuff as a hardened drinker is to alcohol.

Marmalades and Jams

Do you know that jam must be 60 per cent added sugars in order to be called jam? That is the regulation. Unless 60 per cent of the weight of a jar of jam is sugars, it breaks the law. Some of the more health-conscious manufacturers have started to make preserves with half the usual quantity of sugars. They cannot call them just 'jam'. You will find them labelled 'low-sugar preserves', or 'low-sugar jam'. They are thickened with pectin, and contain some preservative, unlike jam, which relies on its 60 per cent sugars for both thickening and preserving. They often contain artificial sweeteners, and have to be refrigerated. But some of these products are really rather a con, because they still contain refined sugars, but often in an unfamiliar form. Many are sweetened with concentrated grape juice (high in fructose), which is really just as refined as concentrated sugar beet juice. In Holland children are busy spooning 'siroop' on to their bread: contents are given as concentrated apple juice and concentrated sugar beet juice. Their parents probably think it is healthier than jam, but the refined sugars content is actually very high. Watch out for such products on the British shop shelves. They are bound to appear sooner or later.

The most expensive preserves of all are usually found in delicatessens and whole food shops. They are made without any added sugars, and must be refrigerated once opened.

'Bread and jam' is a relatively recent invention. The peculiarly British passion for jam started at the turn of the century when sugar became cheaper and fruit production increased. Jam was a good way to preserve and use up surplus fruit. But nowadays we have fridges and freezers. Is jam really the best way to eat fruit? And is bread best eaten covered with sugar? On the whole the British loaf is of such poor quality that it needs something to cover up its appearance and tastelessness. The Italians and Greeks have no need to smother their bread with jam. Better bread needs less jam.

Fruit Juices

Does your day start with a glass of fruit juice? Sweetened or unsweetened? Check the label before you buy it, but remember that fruit juice can have 15 grams added sugar per litre before it must be declared 'sweetened'. There are several unsweetened fruit juices on the market, but many more have had spoonfuls of sugar tipped into them.

Bread

Few breads contain much added sugars. Some of the sweetest are the ones used for wrapping round hamburgers. Eat more bread, but look for good quality.

Cakes, Biscuits

Because cakes, pastries and biscuits are nearly all made with sugars (and fats, salt and white flour), the recommendation is that you eat them less often. If you eat biscuits every day, why not have them every other day instead – but don't eat twice as much to make up for it! Choose the less sweet varieties. Avoid the ones with chocolate or icing on top and filling in the middle. Switching to savoury varieties may not cut down the sugars as much as you think – it is surprising how many savoury biscuits have added sugars. Read the labels carefully. Eat fruit cakes, scones or currant buns instead of the sweeter iced varieties. Better still, avoid cakes and biscuits most of the time and have a sandwich instead. Or why not a piece of fresh fruit? An orange, tangerine, peach, plum, banana. Fruit need not always be an apple. Try to give your children more fruit. Does a fresh peach cost much more than a cake?

Soups, Pickles

Home-made soup usually doesn't contain added sugar, so why does it when you buy it in tins and packets? The original chutneys from India also had no added sugars. It was the British who changed the recipe. Up to one third of the weight of tomato and brown sauces can be sugars. What can we do about it? Apart from making your own pickles, and eating less of the manufactured varieties, not much – except perhaps to write to the manufacturers and ask them why they are drowning the flavour of our food with sugars. The whole point of sauces and pickles was to add interesting taste in the form of spices, herbs and fruits. Sugared tomato sauce poured on to sugared baked beans and sugared peas sounds more like pudding than first course.

Canned Fruit and Vegetables

Some canners have started to produce canned foods without sugars. Until recently, all canned fruit and nearly all vegetables had added sugars. Try the new varieties. If you like them write to the manufacturer and say so. By choosing unsweetened varieties, you will be avoiding an average two teaspoons of sugars for every tin of vegetables, and some five teaspoons in a small tin of fruit!

Yoghurts

All but 7 per cent of the yoghurt eaten in Britain is sweetened. Fruit yoghurts usually contain 5 to 15 per cent sugars or about four teaspoons per carton. They often contain more sugars than fruit. Why not try natural yoghurt with fresh or dried fruit instead?

Desserts are even sweeter. They can be up to 20 per cent sugars; that's one fifth of the carton.

Salads

Five per cent sugar is the average for coleslaw, prawn cocktails, potato salads, mixed vegetables. How long does it take to make your own? All you need is a sharp knife and a good mixture of fresh clean vegetables.

Drinks

A can of Coca-Cola contains about seven teaspoons of sugars, a glass of Lucozade has about eight, a glass of blackcurrant cordial about five, bitter lemon about five per medium bottle, orange squash about two per glass. With the exception of diet drinks and pure fruit juices, most drinks are sweetened. Buy unsweetened fruit juice instead, but check the label first. If you must have them really sweet, choose the ones with artificial sweeteners.

Sweets

It goes without saying that all sweets are on the black list. Eating sweets between meals is worse for your teeth than eating sugar as part of a meal. Give your children a sandwich instead, or a banana, or some dried fruit. Try not to give sweets to babies. If they have never tasted them, they won't weep for them.

In a society where sweets are eaten so often, it is very difficult to say 'no' to all sweets for children. Many parents now give their children all the sweets in one go, which is much better for their teeth than a few sweets eaten more often – but still bad for health. Sweets once a week, followed by a tooth-cleaning session, will do little harm.

Does your children's school have a tuck shop? What are the profits spent on? Many school tuck shops are busy financing such things as sports, entertainments and special events. If you are concerned about the amount of sweets your children eat at school, why not bring the subject up at the Parent-Teacher Association meeting, along with the nutritional quality of school meals? And please don't buy sweets and sweetened drinks for friends and relatives in hospital. Ill people are most in need of highly nourishing food with all their vitamins and minerals intact. There is nearly always room for improvement.

Sugars – A Summary of the Advice

- Eat unsweetened breakfast cereals.

- Stop putting sugar in tea and coffee.

- Eat fewer biscuits and cakes. Choose less sweet varieties.

- Have more fresh fruit, dried fruit or nuts instead.

- Eat less jam, or buy the low-sugar varieties.

- Drink pure fruit juice in preference to fizzy, fruitless sweet squashes and lemonades etc.

- Have fresh fruit instead of sweet puddings.

- Make puddings only occasionally – save time and your children's teeth.

- Read food labels. Look out for the '-ose's.

CHAPTER 9

Milk and Cheese

MILK: HIGH PROTEIN OR HIGH FAT?
BOTTLE TOPS: THE CODE CRACKED.
HARD CHEESE FOR THE CONSUMER.

The Dairy Council would be foolish to ignore the romantic appeal of traditional British country life. Chocolate boxes, seed packets and coffee-table books by the dozen all remind us of our picturesque rural past. Rose-decked cottages, chubby dimpled children, apple-laden trees and frothing dairy churns lovingly tended by blooming dairy maids. This is the stuff that our ancestors' lives were made of. Rural bliss.

Or was it? Painstaking studies by nineteenth-century social pioneers describe a very different picture. Far from living off Daisy's copious quantities of creamy milk and butter, the average Victorian country dwellers scraped a miserable living as best they could. They rarely had enough to eat. Throughout the industrial revolution rural workers were on the whole even more impoverished than workers in the towns. Their living conditions were appalling. Nearly all were severely underweight. Their condition was summed up thus: labourers 'did not live in the proper sense of the word, they merely didn't die' (Canon Girdlestone). Of course this did not apply to everyone. The rich man in his mansion ate well. He it was who dined on legs of lamb and suckling pig, creamy milk and cheese. His poorer workers lived on bread, potatoes, dumplings, and a little pickled pork, treacle and cabbage. Butter, milk and cheese were expensive luxuries which few could afford in anything but tiny amounts.

The idea that the British population has been brought up on great quantities of dairy foods for centuries is quite wrong. Most of the population could not afford them.

The amount of milk, butter, cheese and cream we eat today is far more than in any other century. Every man, woman and child in Britain drinks the equivalent of 4½ pints of milk (as milk, yoghurt and cream), and eats about 4 ozs of cheese and 3½ ozs of butter, each week.

Milk: High Protein or High Fat?

During the twentieth century governments have made strenuous efforts to increase the amount of dairy foods produced. The reason behind this drive towards a milky, buttery diet was partly the very poor physical condition of the mass of the population during the nineteenth and early twentieth centuries. Being the ideal food for infants, milk was considered a perfect food, and nutritionists classified the protein of cow's milk as first-class, because it was so close to the quality of human milk protein when analysed. Several studies in the first half of the twentieth century showed that poor children grew better when given extra milk. In fact, these children were so underfed that they would have grown better given more good food in general.

Of course there is something rather absurd about the notion of a perfect food, for people do not exist on one food alone. Meals consist of a variety of different things. What is lacking in one food should be made up by another. But at the turn of the century, the notion was not quite as absurd as it now seems. The mass of the population lived on a restricted diet. Many of them relied almost entirely on bread and potatoes; theirs was indeed more or less a single-food diet. The idea of supplementing it with one ideal food was reasonable at the time, and the scientists were not aware of the harm that saturated dairy fat can do over a lifetime. Faced with a similar situation today, most nutritionists would opt for more variety: more fresh fruit and vegetables, different kinds of cereals, lean meat and fish. Dairy foods are not essential for health.

Milk was promoted by nutritionists and doctors because of the quality of milk protein. But the protein content is actually rather low. Although the quality of milk protein is closer to that of human milk than any other food, the quantity it provides is small. Milk is about 87 per cent water. Only 3·3 per cent of milk is protein, compared with 9 per cent of bread and 7 per cent of boiled haricot beans. And 3·8 per cent is fat. Milk contains rather more fat than protein. Dairy fats do harm because of the total amount of milk we drink. If we drank very little, it would not matter. And if we drank the same amount of milk as we now do, but with the fat removed, that would not be a problem either. It would be much healthier.

Milk supplies about 13 per cent of the total fat in the average British diet. Furthermore, milk fat is highly saturated and harmful to the arteries. Milk provides 17 per cent of all the saturated fats in our daily food. No other single food provides as much, except butter (14 per cent).

Taken together, dairy foods – milk, cream, butter, cheese – supply 30 per cent of all our fats and 40 per cent of all our saturated fat. If it were not for dairy fats we would all be in better shape.

Not all human societies drink milk. The majority of the world's population gives the habit up in infancy. The Chinese, for example, have no dairy products. They neither drink milk, nor do they eat dairy products. But unfortunately they are learning from Western visitors. Chinese tourist brochures now advertise cow's milk Chinese cheese, produced in southern China for the tourists who presumably cannot manage without it. No doubt the Chinese themselves will soon be polishing off the sweet and sour pork, accompanied by strawberry milkshake, followed by a slice of Chinese cheddar. Most Asian countries were not accustomed to milk until United Nations lorries arrived with boxes full of dried milk powder surplus to EEC and North American requirements. Consuming large amounts of dairy foods is a new habit for mankind.

Finally, the valuable nutrients of milk do not come in the fatty part, but in the watery part underneath. Skimming the fat off the top leaves all the protein and minerals, including calcium, and most of the vitamins. The fat only contains a little vitamin D and vitamin A (apart from fat, that is). We make vitamin D in our skin when we are exposed to sunlight. Most of us have stores in our livers which provide adequate vitamin D in the winter months. The amount of vitamin A in milk is also small: carrots and green vegetables provide far more.

The advantages of drinking full-fat milk are far outweighed by the harm the fat does to our arteries. The nation's children would all have healthier hearts if they were brought up after weaning on low-fat milk instead.

Drinka Pinta Whatta Day

Neighbourhood milkmen sell over 85 per cent of all milk produced. They deal in one major commodity, milk, together with the odd carton of fruit juice or yoghurt. Despite attempts to diversify into other things such as chickens, turkeys, eggs and sweetened drinks, their income still depends on sales of milk. Theirs is largely a single-food trade.

It is therefore remarkable that milkmen are so ignorant about the food they sell. How is it that they sell one main item, and yet are seemingly as unaware and confused as their customers about what the bottle contains? The origin of this strange situation lies not at the feet of the individual roundsmen, but with the Milk Marketing Board, whose chief preoccupation it has been for many years to concentrate our minds on the contents of a silver-top bottle. That is what counts. For silver-top milk is full-cream milk, straight from the churn. What matters is that we drink it. Lots of it. It worries the dairy trade that we drink rather less milk than we used to, and it worries them even more that we might like to have different kinds of low-fat milk available for everyday use. So the advertising and promotion of milk is almost entirely restricted to full-cream liquid milk. If we switched to skimmed milk, it would make the EEC butter mountain even bigger. The farmers would prefer us to drink it instead.

In the summer of 1984 the Milk Marketing Board changed its policy and made fresh pasteurized, semi-skimmed and skimmed milks nationally available: an admirable development. The reason was that low-fat milk had already become generally available in supermarkets; and despite the fact that a lot of it at first was the sterilized or ultra heat treated (UHT) type, with the rather ominous 'Best by' stamp bearing a date of maybe sometime next year, shoppers were buying it in abundance.

Then fresh (pasteurized, not sterilized or UHT) low-fat milk became dramatically more popular in supermarkets; Sainsburys were the first to sell it in large quantities. More recently, St. Ivel's low-fat Shape range has become popular.

So, backed by an advertising campaign suggesting that it was patriotic to buy milk from the roundsman, the Milk Marketing Board is now fighting back. Ask your milkman for semi-skimmed or skimmed fresh pasteurized milk. He may seem confused or unhappy and reach for the first bottle of 'different' milk – such as the rather disgusting sterilized milk or UHT in bottles with metal tops that you have to lever off with old-fashioned openers, or else full-fat homogenized milk (with the red top). He may also tell you the 'sell by' date on low-fat milk is liable to be only one day away; and it does seem that low-fat milk sometimes sits too long on the float. It is odd that we should have to explain to a milkman the difference between the types of milk he sells, but there it is.

The Dutch and the Scandinavians, and many other Europeans, have their milk packaged and bottled in a different way. They have an informed choice. Their milk can be full-fat, half-fat, or no fat. They know what to ask for because milk comes labelled with the quantity of fat it contains.

In Britain most of us are still confused. On the whole, we do not understand the difference between UHT, sterilized, skimmed, homogenized and pasteurized. Until very recently, low-fat milks have been for slimmers only. They have been promoted with tape measures and bikini-clad ladies climbing up the carton. Furthermore, until recently, all these milks have been sterilized, and therefore taste different from the normal pinta. Most of us have been put off skimmed milk as a result. All the indications are that, given the right information, the public is now interested in having healthier milk. Following television programmes in February 1984 about the dangers to our hearts of drinking too much milk fat, the sales of skimmed milk went up 10 per cent in two weeks. Over the last two years, sales of skimmed milk have trebled.

Butter Mountains

Everyone has heard about the butter mountain. But what has caused it?

In 1950 the average European cow produced just 1,500 litres of milk a year. In 1980, the figure was 3,500, and in 1983 it was 5,000, with 8,000 litres envisaged in the future. The increase between 1950 and 1983 is over treble the milk per cow.

EEC rules and regulations are complicated, but what it all boils down to is this. Subsidies paid to a multitude of businesses in agriculture and retailing have encouraged farmers to keep on producing a volume of milk that we, the consumers, do not want to drink. In Britain the Milk Marketing Board is obliged to buy all the milk produced. There is no free market in which over-priced over-producers would go to the wall. Each drop of milk is purchased, at a price set by the government. And milk used in liquid form, for drinking, receives a higher price than milk used for manufacture. The price is controlled and subsidized by government. The Milk Marketing Board is uniquely interested in us the consumers drinking nearly all the milk in full-fat form. What else can they do with it?

If they skim the fat off, who will eat it? We import butter from New Zealand, yet EEC cows are still over-producing milk, and the surplus cream is being piled on to the million tonne butter mountain. There are one million tonnes of skimmed milk sitting in Europe. Nobody wants it. Yet until 1984 our governments continued to buy the milk. We pay for it. Hare-brained schemes are dreamed up to dispose of these heaps of unwanted food. 'Intervention butter' – in other words bits of butter off the top of the mountain – is doled out to charitable institutions and hospitals, where it helps to promote the patients' atherosclerosis. Subsidies come and go. Prices fluctuate. Doorstep delivery men are subsidized to keep our consumption of full-cream milk higher than it otherwise would be. School children are encouraged to help drink up the surplus. All this is controlled by the government. A free market does not operate in the dairy trade.

There are signs that this economic madness may be replaced with a more sensible scheme. For in the summer of 1984, the British government and the EEC both made some small steps towards scaling down the enormous food surpluses within the EEC and also towards conserving the environment. Pressure groups like Friends of the Earth have been saying for years and years that our farming policy is an environmental disaster, as well as an economic fiasco. They have called repeatedly for an end to the destruction of important wildlife sites, which has been encouraged by the EEC and British government subsidies to farmers to maximize food production. Now, at last, it seems the government has got the message. Even the National Farmers' Union are talking about the need for conservation.

The EEC has made steps to cut dairy production, which British farmers say has hit them unfairly. The really unfortunate thing about the way the EEC decided to clobber the dairy industry was the lack of adequate warning to all concerned: suppliers of milking equipment found themselves with cancelled orders overnight; farmers were obliged to reduce the size of their herds within weeks. Yet all of us knew that the production of food surpluses could not go on indefinitely. But even with EEC expenditure cuts in 1984 and 1985, the mountain will not disappear; the system within the EEC is still designed to produce far too much milk.

Fighting the Fat

Without switching to low-fat milks the nation as a whole will find it very difficult to develop healthier arteries. For milk supplies nearly one fifth of all the harmful saturated fat in our diet.

What should you look for in the shops and on the milkman's float? Semi-skimmed and skimmed milk is the answer. But first, here is a guide to all the different kinds of milk sold in Britain.

Milk (Full-fat Milk)

Milk straight from the average British cow contains about 3·8 per cent fat by weight. The level varies slightly from year to year. And the average fat level in any one year is used as a standard, against which next year's milk imports are measured. This is all rather more important to the British dairy trade than you might imagine. For, on the continent, there is a standardization process, with all EEC milk required to have a minimum fat content of 3·5 per cent (not 3·8 per cent). UK and Ireland do not have such a minimum standard for domestic production. But what we *do* have is a regulation which says that no milk can be imported unless it has a fat content of at least a certain amount. And that certain amount is 3·89 per cent for 1984, and 3·88 per cent for 1985. The figure is calculated from the average fat content of the previous year's milk production.

What it all boils down to is that the typical continental pinta with its lower fat content and cheaper price cannot be imported into the UK; a neat little safeguard for the British dairy farmers, and yet one more contributory factor to our high rates of heart attack. The fattiest milk in the EEC, the highest rate of heart disease, both to be found north of the Channel. This full fat milk accounts for nearly 90 per cent of all the milk drunk in Britain.

Even fattier is Channel Islands, Jersey, Guernsey and South Devon milk, with a fat content of at least 4·0, and usually around 4·8 per cent. It can be recognized easily by the rich, yellow, fat which floats on the top of the bottle.

The name 'milk' can *only* be used for full-fat milk. Low-fat milk must be called 'skimmed milk', or 'semi-skimmed milk', according to its fat content. And if anything is added to the milk, the word 'milk' cannot be used in the name. So any low-fat milk for example, which has powdered milk added to it, plus or minus the odd vitamin, must be called something else. Hence Vitapint, the low-fat milk sold by Sainsburys which has added milk solids and vitamins.

Untreated Milk

Raw, untreated (unheated) milk (3·8 per cent fat) comes in bottles with green tops. If the top is green with a gold stripe, the bottle contains raw Channel Islands milk. Very little milk is produced in this way, and the Ministry of Agriculture would like to restrict its distribution. Green-top milk is produced by farms that receive a government licence stating that their herds are brucellosis-free and healthy.

Since the end of April 1985, raw untreated milk is by law only available direct from the producer/retailer. In other words farmers will not be able to sell it through normal distribution channels. The idea is that everyone will then be quite clear what they are buying, because they will have gone out to find it.

Before the common infections of dairy herds were brought under control, and before pasteurization, untreated milk was a major source of infection in Britain. Today, herds are repeatedly treated for serious infections so that the risk from drinking raw milk is very small. However, the Ministry of Agriculture clearly feel that, small though it is, it is still too great, and so they are clamping down on its distribution.

Pasteurized Milk

Nearly all our milk is heat-treated to kill off harmful bacteria. Some bacteria remain in the milk, but they do not cause serious diseases such as brucellosis or tuberculosis. The milk is heated to 63–66 degrees celsius for thirty minutes and then cooled rapidly, or to 72 degrees celsius for fifteen seconds, the high temperature short-time method. Silver-top milk is pasteurized.

Sterilized Milk

An increasing amount of the milk we drink is sterilized. Sterilized milk must be heated to not less than 100 degrees celsius, and the bottles or cartons must be sealed so that the milk is sterile. Ultra-Heat-Treated milk (UHT) has been heated to 132 degrees celsius for not less than one second.

Both these types of milk will keep for several months if sealed. Sterilized or UHT milk has a 'boiled' flavour, which is different from pasteurized. Most people notice the difference when drinking milk on its own. But when it is used in cooking or in tea and coffee, the difference in taste is not so noticeable.

Homogenized milk

Homogenized milk has been agitated or shaken up so that all the fat in the milk is dispersed throughout the liquid in tiny droplets. The cream will not separate and rise to the top of the bottle. (Goats' milk is like this naturally. The fat is in such small droplets that the cream does not separate easily.)

Full-fat and semi-skimmed milk can both be homogenized, because both contain fat. Many people think that homogenized means 'slimming'. It does not. All homogenized milk contains fat. (Without fat there would be nothing to homogenize.)

Semi-skimmed milk

Semi-skimmed milk has had half its fat removed. It contains 1·5 to 1·8 per cent fat. It can be either sterilized or pasteurized. It can be homogenized, although it is not always sold like this. Pasteurized semi-skimmed milk tastes just like silver top with the cream poured off.

Skimmed milk

Skimmed milk has had all its fat removed (less than 0.3 per cent fat remains). It can be either sterilized or pasteurized. Skimmed milk has a rather 'thin' appearance, and a less rich flavour than full-fat milk. When it is used in cooking or in tea and coffee, the difference in flavour is hard to detect.

Bottle Tops and Cartons

More and more milk is now being sold in cartons instead of bottles. And more milk is being bought in supermarkets instead of from the local milkman.

Bottle Tops – The Code Cracked

If you buy milk in bottles, the colours of the tops will tell you what sort of milk they contain. The following colours for milk are laid down by law:

- *Plain green top* – raw, untreated full-fat (3.8 per cent)
- *Green/gold striped top* – raw, untreated full-fat (4.8 per cent) Jersey
- *Plain silver top* – pasteurized full-fat (3.8 per cent)
- *Plain red top* – pasteurized homogenized full-fat (3.8 per cent)
- *Blue/silver striped top* – pasteurized full-fat (3.8 per cent), Kosher for Passover
- *Purple/silver striped top* – pasteurized full-fat (3·8 per cent) Kedassia, Kosher for orthodox Jews

- *Clamped metal top, blue* – sterilized full-fat (3·8 per cent)
- *Clamped metal top, pink* – UHT full-fat (3·8 per cent)

The caps of all milk bottles containing full-fat milk have the 'sell by' date stamped on them. Apart from that, the bottle top need not supply you with any other information. The exception is untreated raw milk, which must be labelled on the top as well as on the bottle itself.

Milk bottles containing full-fat milk must tell you what milk they contain and the name and address of the dairy. However, they are not required to have the fat content stamped on them.

Skimmed and semi-skimmed milk is often sold in cartons, not bottles. However, if it is sold in bottles, the bottle or the top must say 'skimmed milk' or 'semi-skimmed' milk, and whether it is homogenized, pasteurized, sterilized or UHT. The bottle-top colour regulations do not cover skimmed and semi-skimmed milks which can therefore be any colour the dairy cares to choose, except those that are already legally binding (silver, green, red and so on). However, some dairies are now bending the law, using plain coloured tops (like blue or red) for skimmed and semi-skimmed pasteurized milk whose use is by law designated for certain full-fat milks (see above). Others are using striped tops of various colours. To date it seems there is no agreement, although the Dairy Trades Federation is apparently trying to create a voluntary code of practice to standardize colours. Here is another example of how the Ministry of Agriculture have let the industry get themselves, and us, in a muddle. Ask the dairy or your milkman if you see a top you do not recognize. You might be in luck.

The official reason why semi-skimmed and skimmed milks are not covered by the regulations is apparently because most of these milks are sold in cartons rather than bottles; and because so few bottles are involved the dairy trade (the Milk Marketing Board) sees no overwhelming need to control the situation.

Another way of looking at this is that the Milk Marketing

Board is positively discouraging us from buying such milks, by not putting them into easily identifiable bottles and promoting them through doorstep milk deliveries. If we all switched to semi-skimmed milks, that could increase the butter mountain to Himalayan heights. But supermarkets have discovered a large untapped market of people who want to buy healthy food and who have until recently been prevented from doing so by the restrictive practices of many dairies that supply the doorstep delivery floats. Milk bought in supermarkets is easier to carry if it is in a carton rather than a bottle. Hence, the cartons.

Cartons

If you buy your milk in cartons, look for the words 'skimmed (or semi-skimmed) pasteurized milk'.

Some supermarkets now sell fortified milks. Vitapint, for example, is skimmed or semi-skimmed milk to which extra dried milk solids have been added to give it a bit more body. Extra vitamins are also added. It tastes slightly different from other pasteurized milk because of the added vitamins and milk powder.

Milk Labelling: The Missing Information

At the moment there is no legislation that requires dairies to inform their customers in writing about the exact fat content of their bottles or cartons. Such information would give us all more freedom of choice. We would know if the milk was $4 \cdot 8$, $3 \cdot 8$, $1 \cdot 8$, or less than $0 \cdot 3$ per cent fat by weight.

The Dairy Trades Federation produced a document in 1984 which said that nutritional labelling of dairy foods would soon begin. The document represented the consensus of agreement amongst dairy trades; therefore it was the 'lowest common denominator' type of document. It said that milk would soon be labelled with total fats, not with saturated fats. Put like this, milk looks rather good. Total fats, $3 \cdot 8$ per cent. Not much, is it? But remember that milk is nearly 90 per cent water. And also that milk fat is about 60 per cent saturated; and we drink a lot of it (4 pints a week) so the amount of saturated fat we get from it is large. Fat supplies 53 per cent of calories in milk, and over half of that fat is saturated. (The remaining 47 per cent of calories come from protein and lactose carbohydrate.) The Dairy Trades Federation might have been hoping to look responsible, at least in the eyes of MAFF. For if the industry goes ahead with this voluntary labelling, albeit of a minimal kind, then maybe MAFF will put off the day when more extensive labelling legislation is brought in. Many branches of the food industry are now doing the same thing; trying hard to convince their retailers and MAFF civil servants that labelling with total fat (per cent of total weight) is all that is necessary. Anything else, like fats or saturated fats (as a per cent of calories) or total added sugars, or polyunsaturated fats, would be too confusing for the consumer, who is apparently too stupid to understand, or too busy to be interested. Does that sound like you?

Milk Not From Cows

In response to the demand for slimming products, and to increased public belief that vegetable fat or oil must be healthier than animal fat, several coffee whiteners have been produced. Coffee Mate for example, is made of glucose syrup, vegetable oils and milk solids. It is 34 per cent fat, and that fat is 98 per cent saturated. It is much more saturated than full-cream milk.

Other non-dairy whiteners are often high in saturated fat. Although they may be based on skimmed milk powder, saturated vegetable fats may be added to them.

Stick to dried skimmed milk instead of these products. It is much healthier.

Goat's Milk
Goat's milk contains 4·5 per cent fat. Many people think that

goat's milk is healthier than cow's. Certainly some people are allergic to cow's milk, and for them goat's milk may be a useful alternative, as it does not appear to produce the same allergic response.

But the fat in goat's milk is predominantly saturated: 69 per cent, compared with 61 per cent in cow's milk. And without the right machinery it is difficult to remove the fat from goat's milk because it is so finely dispersed through the liquid. Little of it rises to the top of the bottle.

A word of warning: goat's milk is just as unsuitable for small babies as cow's milk, unless it has been modified to reduce the protein content. If you have a baby who appears to be allergic to cow's milk, get proper advice from a dietitian about safe alternatives.

Yoghurt

Low fat yoghurt is a healthy alternative to cream and can be used in cooking to thicken sauces (do not boil it or it will curdle).

Beware the amount of added sugars in fruit and flavoured yoghurts. Fresh fruit is a healthier sweetener.

Greek-style yoghurts tend to be thicker and creamier and, because they have been drained, may have a higher fat content. Some are as much as ten per cent fat, compared with low fat varieties which are less than one per cent.

Hard Cheese for the Consumer

While milk consumption has been gradually falling from an all-time high in 1951, cheese consumption has been increasing. In 1980, we ate 37 per cent more cheese than in 1955. The fat content of cheeses varies a great deal. It all depends on how they are made, and how much water they contain.

Many continental cheeses contain less fat than British ones. This is because they contain more water; the fat is more diluted. But the labels on French cheese are deceptive. They tell you the amount of fat in the dry matter of the cheese, which makes cheeses such as Brie and Camembert seem extremely fatty. On a dry-weight basis, they are 40 to 50 per cent fat (which is how they are labelled), whereas on a wet-weight basis (which is how you eat them) they are about 25 per cent fat.

Below is a list of the fat content of some of the more popular cheeses.

CHEESE	FAT CONTENT g/100 g
Brie	26
Caerphilly	31
Camembert	27
Cheddar	33
cheese spread	23
Cheshire	32
Cottage, natural	4
Cottage, flavoured	3-5
cream	47
Curd cheese (Ricotta)	5-10
Danish Blue	30
Double Gloucester	32
Edam	25
Gouda	30
Leicester	32
Lymeswold	40
Mozzarella	25
Parmesan	30
processed	25
Sage Derby	33
Shape Cheese	16
Stilton	40
Tendale	50
Wensleydale	31

When you buy cheese, buy the more mature ones, which are stronger and have a better flavour. You may need less, particularly in cooking.

The quality of British cheese has gone noticeably downhill in the last thirty years. Industrial methods of cheese-making produce wetter cheeses that are less mature than the traditionally produced 'farmhouse' varieties. (The word 'farmhouse' does not necessarily indicate that the cheese has been produced by traditional maturation methods.)

The 'real cheese' movement is now starting to catch on, and with luck it may have the same success as the 'Real Ale' movement over the last few years.

Most of us taste real cheese only rarely. The plastic-wrapped varieties on the shop shelves are a far cry from their traditional counterparts. There is high politics behind the disappearance of traditional and varied British cheeses, all to do with the restrictive selling practices of the Milk Marketing Board. The Board does not like dealing in small quantities of milk, so the small dairies lose out.

Visit your local Italian, Greek and delicatessen shops. Some whole food shops sell a variety of British cheeses not found in supermarkets. Ask what is available. Goat's and sheep's cheeses are now produced in quite large quantities in Britain. Small dairies are trying to make a comeback in Britain, producing their own distinctive varieties, but they need our full support if they are to survive.

Better quality cheeses do cost more, but if the flavour is well developed you will not use such large amounts.

The habit of eating bread and cheese with butter is peculiar to the North Europeans, and is a modern habit. Far healthier is to do as the French and Mediterranean people do – leave the butter out altogether. Bread (and butter) are discussed elsewhere in this book. But remember that butter is a highly saturated fat. No less than 60 per cent of it is saturated. It supplies 10 per cent of all the fat we eat and 14 per cent of the saturated fat.

Milk and Cheese: A Summary of the Advice

- Buy skimmed or semi-skimmed, fresh, pasteurized milk.
- Use skimmed milk in cooking.
- Give your children semi-skimmed milk when they are weaned on to a mixed diet. But never give skimmed or full-fat unmodified cow's milk to babies under 6 months old.
- If your child has milk at school, ask the school if they will provide skimmed milk.
- Ask canteens to provide skimmed milk for tea and coffee.
- Write to your local dairy if your milkman offers no choice.
- Choose better quality mature cheese.
- Use stronger cheese for cheese sauces.
- Eat more low- and medium-fat cheeses.
- Yoghurt is a good alternative to cream.

CHAPTER 10

Vegetables

WEARY CABBAGE AND TIRED TURNIPS. SQUEEZE BUT COOK GENTLY.
LETTUCE IS NOT ENOUGH. BEANS AND GAS.
THE CASE OF THE DISAPPEARING SPUD. PESTICIDES.

As far as good cooking is concerned, one of the most attractive
recommendations for good health is to increase the amount of
vegetables we eat. This, probably more than anything else,
could improve our culinary standards, for a wide variety of
vegetables cooked in a healthy way is the basis of all the world's
great cuisines. The success of Far Eastern, Indian, Middle
Eastern, Mediterranean and French cooking depends on a
supply of fresh vegetables in prime condition, cooked with
imagination, skill and good quality oils, herbs and spices.

The British have never been very good with vegetables.
Cookery books written over 100 years ago describe how green
leafy vegetables should be boiled not once but several times in
copious quantities of well-salted water. Then they were
smothered in butter or thick sauces.

Nor have salads ever been our strong point. For too many
people, 'salad' means a couple of flabby lettuce leaves, two
slices of cucumber and half a tomato, all drowned in thick salad
dressing made of tasteless oil, bad quality vinegar, sugar and
salt.

Creating new and healthy vegetable dishes is a challenge for canteens, hospital kitchens, restaurants and the majority of British households. A greater variety of vegetables is available than ever before. All we need to do is to learn how to cook them.

Potatoes came from Peru, peppers and tomatoes from Mexico, globe artichokes from the native Americans, carrots from Afghanistan, cucumbers from India, runner beans from Latin America, marrows from the USA, onions and aubergines from Asia, celery and broccoli from Italy, lettuce and peas from the Near East. Whatever did the British eat before these vegetables were imported? Broad beans, beets and cabbage were our Iron Age stand-bys. We cannot even claim spinach as our own. That came from Nepal.

Many of the vegetables we now eat were introduced from the sixteenth century onwards, although many vegetables that were common in the Middle Ages have now disappeared. Some of the new ones, like aubergines and green peppers, have only very recently been grown here. Even tomatoes were not grown in commercial quantities until the twentieth century.

Having imported the vegetables, we are now in the process of importing the cooking to go with them. Methods of cooking and serving vegetables described in today's most enlightened cookery books are completely different from those of the 1950s. Cooking time has got shorter and shorter; the potful of boiling water has evaporated; the bicarbonate has gone; garlic, ginger and fresh herbs have appeared. Vegetable dishes are being transformed.

In part, we have to thank our resident ethnic minority communities. Asians, Cypriots, Chinese and West Indians have introduced us to new vegetables and to new ways of dealing with them. We now eat all kinds of plants in salads that many would have shunned only thirty years ago. Some of us still blanch at the sight of raw fennel and cabbage, but the message is slowly getting through. Coleslaw, albeit in its most dreadful form, can now be eaten in hospital canteens where a few years ago warm lettuce would have been the only raw vegetable available.

Weary Cabbage and Tired Turnips

Despite the ever-increasing variety of vegetables available to us, the amount of fresh vegetables we eat is declining steadily. In 1981 we ate just 12 oz of fresh green vegetables each week, and 16 oz of other fresh vegetables, not including potatoes.

Now 12 plus 16 equals 28, which makes just 4 oz a day. Think what that might look like: the odd onion, a couple of carrots, a few sprouts. The amount is pathetic.

In addition we eat a little less than ½ oz of frozen vegetables, half of which are peas. On top of that comes less than 1½ oz of tinned vegetables, half of which are baked beans. The grand total is 6 oz a day. A miserable quantity.

The Scots barely manage to get through 1 oz of fresh green vegetables each day. Then come Northerners and the Welsh. At the top of the league are the inhabitants of the south-west, who top 2 oz of fresh greenery per day. Green-fingered with our gardens we may be; in our kitchens we fail.

With all that horticulture and technology can offer us, why are vegetables so unpopular? One third of the vegetables we eat are cabbage and peas. The variety found in the street markets of London and the biggest cities has not reached the rest of the country. Visit a greengrocer in the Welsh valleys or Scotland and what do you find? Half-dead cabbage, swedes, turnips, parsnips, flabby spring greens. Where are the peppers, ladies' fingers, aubergines, Chinese leaves, celery, spinach, chicory, iceberg lettuces, fresh ginger, coriander, parsley and watercress?

Who promotes fresh vegetables? The amount of money spent on advertising fresh food is minute by comparison with what goes on frozen peas, baked beans and crisps. When did you last see an advertisement for home-made vegetable soup or salad?

When it comes to advertising, fresh vegetables are an irrelevant part of our diet. They are not worth it. The profit margin on a packet of frozen peas or a tin of tomato soup is far greater than that on a bunch of watercress.

Fibre, Vitamins and Minerals

All vegetables contain dietary fibre, of which we eat too little for good health. Vegetable fibre, like that of whole grain cereals and fruit, speeds the passage of food through the intestine. The more fibre in the diet, the faster food travels, the bigger the stools produced, and the softer they become (see also page 14). Our diet lacks sufficient vegetables, which is one reason why, as a nation, we are constipated.

Vegetables do other things in the intestine besides speeding up transit. They fuel the colonic gas works. Bacteria live in the colon (large intestine) and set to work there on the digested products that arrive from the 22 feet of the small intestine and stomach.

The food we eat spends less than eight hours travelling through the stomach and small intestine. By far the greater part of its time inside us is spent in the colon.

Food containing little fibre leaves little residue after digestion in the small intestine: the amount entering the colon is small. In contrast, food containing a lot of fibre results in large quantities of residue being tipped into the top of the colon.

This is what happens if the colon is regularly filled up with fibrous material. The fibre provides food for the bacteria which inhabit the colon. The more food they are delivered, the faster the bacteria grow and multiply. There is a ferment of activity. Large numbers of bacteria retain fluid within the system. As the digested material travels down the colon, it remains soft and fluid. It produces large, soft stools at frequent intervals. The whole system is operating at speed.

If, on the other hand, there is very little fibre in food, just the opposite happens. Tiny quantities of residue dribble into the top of the colon. Not much material here for the bacteria to bother about. Little residue, few bacteria, small bulk. Little water is retained within the system. The faeces formed are small and hard, with the consistency of firm clay. There are few of them. Their production is a rare event.

British meals spend about 70 or 80 hours inside us, and only about eight of them are in the stomach and small intestine. Our food makes its way through six feet of colon in three days! By contrast, food fairly plummets through the system in rural Africa: it takes about half a day to travel the entire length of the digestive tract.

Dietary fibre also gives rise to what in polite circles is known as flatulence or indigestion. In simpler language, it produces gas. It is extremely bad manners to draw attention to this problem. Witness the consternation in a crowded room when the unmentionable happens. A roomful of people do their best to disown the surrounding air. Maybe we will have to change our manners! Vegetables in particular produce gas in the colon. Cabbage, the old British favourite, is one of the worst offenders.

Vitamin C is a familiar nutrient to most people, but folic acid is less widely known. Folic acid (folate), one of the B vitamins, is found in green leafy vegetables.

Many people in Britain consume only the bare minimum of vitamin C and the average amount of folic acid eaten is actually about half the internationally recommended level.

Vitamin C deficiency results in tiredness, weakness, irritability, depression, muscle and joint pains, loss of weight and bleeding gums. Blood vessels lose their firmness, and little red spots appear under the skin where the tiny blood capillaries have broken. Elderly people sometimes develop this condition because they eat insufficient fresh fruit and green vegetables. Vitamin C deficiency is probably much more common in Britain than we realize, due mainly to the small amount of fresh plant food we eat and also because of the way it is cooked.

Government analyses of the average British diet show it to be deficient in folic acid. The fewer fresh green vegetables eaten, the lower the folic content of the diet. Deficiency causes anaemia, which results in inefficient circulation of oxygen in the blood. It produces tiredness, depression and irritability, and can lead to mental deterioration.

There is also a strong evidence that lack of folic acid is a cause of neural tube defects (spina bifida and other disorders) in babies. Mothers whose diet before conception and in very early pregnancy is low in this vitamin run a greater risk of having a baby with this problem. The UK has the highest rate of neural tube defects in Europe.

Heat and storage destroy both vitamin C and folic acid. Newly picked green vegetables contain large amounts of both vitamins, but the longer they sit about in containers, the lower the vitamin content becomes. Flabby green leaves may retain only a fraction of the original quantity. Other good sources of folic acid are liver, lean meats, and wholemeal bread.

The human body is designed to take in large amounts of potassium and small amounts of sodium. Fresh vegetables of all kinds contain large amounts of potassium and other essential minerals and little sodium. But this balance of nature is destroyed by the British diet, very high in sodium, low in vegetables and thus in potassium. The result is a population at risk of high blood pressure. We need to eat lots of lightly cooked vegetables. And the less water they are boiled in, the less minerals go down the sink.

Squeeze But Cook Gently

Freshness is of paramount importance, both for flavour and nutritional value. If you can pick your own vegetables from the garden, so much the better. Generally their flavour will not be rivalled by commercial varieties grown by intensive methods.

Avoid vegetables that look limp and crumpled. Even though soaking their stalks in water wakes them up a little, they are of inferior quality to really fresh vegetables.

Be particular. As a rule the British public is not allowed to inspect fresh food too closely, which is considered to be a strange continental habit. But why pay for a bagful of poor quality food? Make sure the vegetables you buy are in prime condition.

The standard of vegetable cooking in British institutions has a reputation for being generally unrivalled in its awfulness. The vat of salted water goes on to boil at 10.30 a.m. The vegetables come out of the freezer and begin to simmer at 11.00 a.m. Lunch is served from 12 until 2.00. The vegetables are uneatable.

Unfortunately many households do little better. Too many children are brought up to think that cabbage begins to cook an hour in advance of the meal. Saucepans of water, salt, bicarbonate of soda to retain some semblance of greenness: the final product is a culinary and nutritional disaster. You can tell the areas of Britain that specialize in this particular branch of cookery by the packets of dried peas in the shops: they all contain a little bag of bicarbonate of soda. The manufacturers know their customers' habits.

However, these archaic practices are slowly declining, and not before time, for many people have probably never tasted the true flavour of fresh vegetables. They do not know what they are missing.

Many hospitals around the country, and also many works canteens, have recently had a major re-think about the meals they supply, and the way in which they are cooked. Vegetables in particular are being given priority, because they are both healthy and delicious when properly cooked. In the interests of their customers' health, caterers and cooks, encouraged by nutritionists and dietitians, are slowly revising their menus. If you eat meals regularly in a canteen and think things could be improved, you might give your views to the chief cook.

Vegetable cookery in Japan and other Eastern countries is very different. Few vegetables are boiled. Many are steamed, or cooked in a wok. Each vegetable is cooked with precision, for time is of the essence to preserve flavour.

Wok cookery is simple. You can buy a large wok cheaply in most Chinese supermarkets, and also in most kitchen shops. They are large round-bottomed circular pans, about a foot in diameter and about four inches deep.

Put a tiny bit of oil in the bottom and cook the vegetables for only a few seconds or minutes over a hot flame, moving them around as they cook in their own juice. This produces crisp vegetables very different from boiled peas and cabbage. All kinds of vegetables, roots and leaves, can be cooked in a wok, but each requires a different length of time in the pan. Buy or borrow a Chinese cookery book and find out how to do it.

Vegetables to be cooked by this method should be cut up into pieces with a large surface area. In other words, it is best to cut a carrot into thin strips rather than round chunks. The larger the surface area in comparison with its size, the shorter the cooking time needed. Large chunks are over-cooked on the outside by the time the middle is ready.

Many vegetables make their own juice while cooking. Leeks and spinach, for example, shed water as they cook, so it is not necessary to add any before you start. A tiny bit of oil in the saucepan will stop them burning at the beginning. A firm lid retains the moisture, and they cook in their own steam. They have most flavour while still bright in colour.

If you boil vegetables, use as little water as possible and boil it before you put the vegetables in. Take them out when they are still firm. Use the juice to make soups, sauce or gravy.

Steamed cabbage has a much better flavour than boiled. Again, Chinese shops sell steamers, the bamboo variety that can be stacked one on top of the other. Kitchen shops sell stainless-steel steamers that can be used in saucepans of any size or shape; they expand to fill the space. Steamed vegetables have far more flavour than their boiled counterparts.

Do vegetables need salt? Well, it all depends on how they are cooked. Over-boiled vegetables certainly lack something, with or without salt. But it is surprising how much more tasty vegetables become when cooked with care, for a short time. Their own flavour is more pronounced. And there are plenty of alternative flavours to salt. Spinach, for example, is delicious served with a little olive oil and fresh lemon juice. Green beans are very good with garlic. Many people are surprised to discover that vegetables without salt are actually very good indeed.

Lettuce Is Not Enough

Salads can be made with almost any vegetable. The variety is limitless. Lettuce, cucumber and tomatoes are the British favourites, but these vegetables are no good for year-round use. Cucumbers and tomatoes are expensive in winter. Tomatoes are quite tasteless when grown at commercial speed in hot-houses. They need sun and slow growth to develop their full flavour. A shop tomato is never as good as the one you grow yourself. Lettuces are usually a poor vegetable in winter: expensive and heartless.

Adapt your recipes to the vegetables in season: carrots, red and white cabbage, fennel, peppers, potatoes, beans of all kinds, nuts, fruit, watercress – salad can be made with anything. But it can be wrecked with poor quality salad dressing.

Many commercial salad creams contain sugar; nearly all contain salt. They are usually made with cheap vinegar, and you are not always told which oil has been used. Why not make your own? It only takes a couple of minutes. Try fresh lemon juice instead of vinegar, and use fresh herbs and less salt. Use good quality oils for salads: it really is worth it. Olive and sesame oil both have distinctive flavours that are delicious used with the right vegetables. You can also make salad dressings with low-fat yoghurt instead of oils.

If you see a vegetable you do not know, ask what it is. Try it.

Invest in a few cookery books on world cookery, and you will be able to find out how to use it. Between them Chinese, Japanese, Indian, Middle Eastern, Italian and French cooking should come up with a recipe.

It is often best to use cookery books for reference rather than for cast-iron rules. For example, many French recipes, particularly from northern France, rely heavily on butter. Parts of the recipe are healthy, others not so. Japanese cooking involves large quantities of soya sauce, which is very salty. On the other hand, it can teach you a lot about developing the full flavour of food. Extract what is healthy from a variety of different sources.

Beans and Gas

Beans have a reputation for producing flatulence. Surely these things are no good for the average inhibited British consumer! But every week each of us eats a quarter of a large tin of baked beans: 4 oz per week.

Apart from that our bean record is not healthy. We only eat ½ oz per week of other kinds of dried beans, and sales of canned beans other than the baked variety are very low.

Beans are one of the healthiest foods. Low in saturated fat, high in dietary fibre, protein and minerals, beans are a staple food for most of the world. Together with cereals, they are the basis of the predominantly vegetarian diet on which most of the world lives.

Beans and cereals keep Africans, Chinese, Indians and Mexicans alive. Not just alive; they also keep them in good health. Their intestines are in better shape than ours because beans provide very large amounts of dietary fibre. The baked bean may save British colons from going on strike altogether!

Britain needs more beans.

One reason why we are not too keen on using dried beans may be that cookery books advise you to soak them overnight or for twenty-four hours. That means you have to plan your meals at least a day in advance.

However, many beans need no soaking at all. Brown lentils and black-eye beans, for example, can be cooked (without soaking) in under 1 hour. Yellow or orange lentils cook in under half an hour.

Other beans take longer. But instead of several hours of soaking, pour boiling water over them and leave them for about three quarters of an hour before cooking. Alternatively, put beans straight in to cook. In a pressure cooker, most will be cooked within one hour.

Make sure that beans are properly cooked. They need not be mushy, but they should not be hard in the middle, because a few contain toxins when raw. If they are brought to the boil, heat will kill these poisons. Raw beans are also indigestible and produce flatulence.

Throw away the soaking water. If you have not soaked the beans, throw away the boiling water after they have been cooking for about fifteen minutes and replace it with fresh water. This removes some of the chemicals in the skin of the bean that cause flatulence.

Baked beans are very popular. They are Britain's most successful canned food, and one of the healthiest processed foods available, despite the fact that they contain added sugars and added salts. The quantity of sugars added is now a matter of dispute. The official HMSO book *The Composition of Foods* (1978) which gives nutritional analysis of about 1,000 foods, says baked beans contain 5·2 per cent sugars but Heinz baked beans on sale in Greece in September 1984 had an extra label (in Greek) declaring a very different sugar content. These baked beans were manufactured in England (it said on the label "made in England H. J. Heinz Co. Ltd, Hayes, Middx. U84 8AL"). Having found their way to Greece, they acquired a new sticky label to cover the original list of ingredients, and that label said "ZAXAPH (sugar) 15%." Then it gave the telephone number of the Heinz representative in Athens:

3218788. The value of 5·2 per cent, widely quoted in books and magazines and derived from the official handbook, would appear to have been used on analyses of baked beans done some years ago. So what is the correct figure? How much better it would be for consumers if the precise quantity of each ingredient were written clearly on the label (in English!).

Baked beans with fish fingers is many children's favourite dish, and a much healthier meal than fried sausages or greasy hamburgers. If children gave up most of the rest of the sugars they eat, the amount they get from baked beans would be much less important.

If you are offered a choice of baked beans or sausage, or Spam, or corned beef, or fatty mince, go for the baked beans every time. But if you cook them yourself, you can make a healthier and tastier dish.

Most supermarkets now sell a few different beans: haricot, kidney beans, chick peas, yellow and green lentils, split peas, brown beans. But some whole food shops sell a much larger variety.

You do not have to be a cranky vegetarian to use beans in cooking. Use them in stews to spread out the meat. They are much cheaper.

Hummus, a Middle Eastern speciality, is becoming very popular in Britain. It is made of ground chick-peas, lemon, garlic and sesame paste. Eaten with bread and salad, it is a perfect healthy meal. Hummus is very easy to make if you have a blender. And other kinds of beans can be prepared in a similar way to make a delicious start to the meal.

Beans do not always have to be hot. Why not use them in salads? Mix them with salad vegetables if you do not like them on their own. Try new recipes.

The Case of the Disappearing Spud

For the last 30 years enough potatoes have been grown in Britain to provides everybody with 4½ lb a week.

However, household purchases show a different picture. In 1955 we ate nearly 4 lb of fresh potatoes per week at home. In 1980 we ate less than 2½ lb. So if the same amount of potatoes is being produced, where have all the rest of the potatoes gone? The case of the disappearing spud.

Take a look at some foods in the supermarket, and you will find the answer. Crisps, potato rings, potato sticks, instant mash; potato starch even finds its way into ice cream.

If you were running a crisp factory, this is how your potato balance sheet would work out. Take 1,000 lb of potatoes. Remove 100 lb in peeling, 27 lb in trimming, 18 lb in slicing, add 82 lb of oil and flavouring, lose 667 lb in cooking, and you will finish up with 270 lb of crisps. This is what the food industry calls 'added value'.

What has been added? Flavour and fat, and salt. More important, what has been taken away? Peel, water, vitamin C, dietary fibre.

But added value has nothing to do with nutritional value. That doesn't come into it. Added value means the addition of *economic* value – in other words, profit. Peeling, trimming, frying, flavouring, packaging, advertising, distributing – all these processes require machinery and provide jobs. Picked and sold to the consumer, 1,000 lb of potatoes produce few jobs and use little machinery. Turned into just 270 lb of crisps, they work an economic miracle. And that is why the Ministry of Agriculture are so keen on such products. They provide employment, engineering, advertising, distribution networks that the humble potato on its own could not rival. A pound of potato crisps costs forty or fifty times more than a pound of potatoes.

Since the last war, we have been eating an increasing number of potato-based products and fewer whole potatoes. In nutritional terms, 'subtracted value' would be an apt description. Potatoes are a valuable part of the diet because of their starch and their fibrous material, found throughout the potato but particularly in the peel. Potatoes are also a cheap source of vitamin C, although peeled potatoes contain much less than unpeeled ones.

Fatty potato products have lost their water and much of their fibrous material. They have lost their vitamin C. They have soaked up fats and have been covered with salt. They are easy to eat. A packet of crisps is not very filling. It's probably the quantity of salt that stops you in the end, not the volume of the food.

How to Cook Potatoes

Potatoes are healthy food. It all depends on how they are cooked. And for flavour, it all depends on the variety. For although there are over 350 varieties in the UK, only about half a dozen of them appear on greengrocers' stalls and in the supermarkets. There is now a regulation that potatoes must be labelled with their variety, so you know what you are being offered. Most of us have seen King Edwards, Désirée, and Maris Piper. But how about Purple Congo, Lumper, Salad Blue, Kerrs Pink, Arran Banner or Doon Star? The problem is that of all the potatoes produced in Britain, almost half find their way into food processing. Between them, farmers and manufacturers want a high yield, disease resistant, uniform shape (for peeling machines),uniform colour, good slicing and frying quality, which all go together to produce an article consistent in taste, appearance and smell. In fact, taste is really rather irrelevant; at least as far as the potato goes, the less taste the better. For most of these products are sliced and then sprayed with concoctions of artificial flavours. Far better that a strong natural flavour does not interfere. So crisps are usually made of Record variety, and frozen chips of Pentland Dell.

If you are interested in trying different potato varieties, you will probably have to grow them yourself. So you could invest some time talking to local gardening enthusiasts, and you may eventually find something interesting.

Boiled potatoes retain more vitamin C if cooked unpeeled.

Steamed have more flavour. They are very good steamed with a onion or two, and some herbs. Yoghurt makes a good sauce with chives or spring onions.

Do mashed potatoes always need butter? What about plain yoghurt and parsley instead? Or a little olive oil and freshly ground pepper? Or just milk. Add less salt.

Try alternative fillings to butter. Quark (a very low-fat cheese) or curd cheese and chives; a sprinkle of Parmesan; yoghurt and herbs. Visit the baked potato shops that are springing up all over the place for a healthier snack than hot dogs or hamburgers. A baked potato doesn't always have to swim in butter. Eaten with a stew, it may need nothing except the juice from the pot.

Eat roast potatoes and chips less often. Fry them in vegetable oil (corn, soya, sunflower, safflower, etc). If you cut potatoes into small pieces, they soak up more fat; floury potatoes rather than the firmer varieties do so too. So use firm potatoes, cut into larger chunks. The chips you make at home will be healthier than those you can buy from chip shops, if you use good oil.

PESTICIDES: POISONS TO INSECTS – AND US?

What about pesticides? A good question. Very sensibly, many people ask whether the advice to eat more fruit, vegetables and cereals is really as good as it sounds. What's the point in studiously avoiding sugars, saturated fats and processed starches, if only to be confronted with a large plateful of plant foods which quite possibly are contaminated with traces of harmful chemicals?

In 1984 the *Journal* of the Association of Public Analysts published the results of the analyses of pesticide residues in 178 vegetable and cereal samples, and 305 soft fruit samples. The Association of Public Analysts is an independent and highly respected organization. Their survey revealed that 61 samples of vegetables (one third) had detectable residues, and of these 37 (one fifth) were at or above the acceptable limit. Of the 305 fruit samples, 103 (one third) were contaminated. The pesticides involved were DDT on blackcurrants, apples and lettuce, aldrin on mushrooms, dimethoate on cherries, gooseberries, peas, plums and mushrooms, and mevinphos on cherries.

The Association of Public Analysts were rightly very concerned at the results. Pesticides are poisons, by definition. Most of them are harmful to a wide range of species, both plant and animal. The extent of the damage they do to humans both as individual pesticides, and in combination first with each other, and second with other constituents or additives in food, is usually not well understood.

Most of the food we eat has probably at some time been in contact with pesticides. Fruits, vegetables and cereals, and meat, via animal feed, are all likely to contain at least traces of different pesticides. Therefore it is reasonable to ask how a pesticide manufacturer goes about putting a new product on the market: how much information does the general public have about the safety both to humans and to the rest of the environment of existing or new pesticides; and how well controlled are the levels of pesticides in foodstuffs?

The Pesticide Safety Precaution Scheme (PSPS) is a formal voluntary agreement between the pesticides industry and government, whereby pesticides are given clearance for use in the UK. The pesticide manufacturers submit their own test data to the government, and the PSPS committees decide whether the product is safe for humans, livestock, domestic animals, beneficial insects, wildlife and the environment. Manufacturers have undertaken that no pesticide will be introduced in the UK without prior approval from PSPS.

Second, manufacturers can submit test data to the Ministry of Agriculture, Fisheries and Food to demonstrate that their product does indeed do what it claims to do, and thereby gain

'Approval'. But manufacturers can and do sell pesticide products in the UK without 'Approval'.

This voluntary (that is, non-statutory) system has worked well for over twenty-five years, according to the Ministry of Agriculture. But such a system cannot be successful in all respects. The experimental test data submitted to PSPS is derived from experiments conducted by the pesticide companies themselves, and is confidential. It is not routinely available for scrutiny by the general public. Pressure groups such as Friends of the Earth concerned for the future of the environment have been refused sight of this data. It is not suggested that all pesticide manufacturers supply PSPS with phoney data. However, it is questionable whether all pesticide manufacturers, civil servants and political parties have at the forefront of their minds the protection of rare butterflies, bees and birds, and the desire to remove all traces of harmful chemical residues from the food chain.

The Banned Poisons Allowed in Britain

Pesticides currently on sale in the UK contain some extremely nasty ingredients. Seven of these give particular cause for concern, because they are probably either carcinogenic, teratogenic, mutagenic, skin irritants or nerve poisons, being harmful to humans, animals, birds or other 'non-pest' species. They are dichlorvos, dieldrin, aldrin, thiram, captan, aldicarb, and 2, 4, 5-T. There are 170 pesticide products containing these ingredients on sale in the UK, destined for use in forestry, on food crops, in homes and in gardens. These seven ingredients have been banned or severely restricted in many countries, yet in the UK they are still on widespread sale. Why?

As far as the level of pesticide residues in food is concerned, the government routinely monitors levels in national food samples, and is satisfied that average levels are generally below accepted maximum residue limits adopted by the United

Nations. However, as the survey conducted by the Public Analysts reveals, many foodstuffs are well above the limits. The weakness of the present system is that the precise location of harmful contamination is not traced back. Furthermore, surveillance is not widespread. Environmental Health Offices need more money and time to make a thorough job of surveillance.

Nobody can ever be sure that every foodstuff is free from all pesticide contamination. Some pesticides persist in the soil for years; in addition, if the farmer next door sprays, wind blows the pesticide on to neighbouring areas. Pesticides are a matter of public concern, and better controls are necessary. And it is outrageous that information about the safety of the environment and our food is kept secret from us. We are entitled to full information about what goes into our food: the quantities and precise definition of ingredients, additives and contaminants.

If you are concerned, write to shop managers, asking them what precautions they are taking to safeguard their customers. Write to your MP, Euro MP, or local councillors. Write to food manufacturers.

Meanwhile, eating vegetables is not likely to increase your risk. Vegetables destined for canning, freezing or fresh sale are all equally likely to be treated with pesticides.

Looking to the future, the Food and Environment Protection Bill (on its way through Parliament at the time of writing) is a step in the right direction towards curtailing the unnecessary and harmful use of excessive pesticide application. However, it is only an 'enabling' bill, which will empower ministers to release information to the public and lay down statutory limits for contamination of foods. There is *no guarantee* that these powers will be used. They may simply gather dust in Whitehall.

Vegetables – A Summary of the Advice

- Eat more vegetables of all kinds.
- Eat more salads.
- Cook green vegetables for a shorter time in less water.
- Use less salt, and more alternative flavourings.
- Eat more beans and potatoes.
- Protest about pesticides.

CHAPTER 11

Fruit and Nuts

TRIFLES AND TELEPHONES. PIP-PIP TO THE PITMASTON PINE APPLE.
ADIEU TO FLAVOUR. DRIED AND CANNED FRUIT, AND JUICE.
EAT FRESH FRUIT AND NUTS AS SNACKS.

The British eat less fresh fruit than almost any other
Europeans. Our total consumption comes to a miserable 2½
oz of fresh fruit per day. Lowest of all are the Northerners at 2
oz; highest are the Londoners: 3½ oz. These are the quantities
we buy to eat at home. Even taking account of the fruit we eat
in canteens and elsewhere, the daily total is very low: less than
the equivalent of one medium-sized apple.

What is wrong with fresh fruit? Why don't we like it much?
The population seems to be having some difficulty shaking off
the attitudes and habits of earlier generations.

Scurvy, caused by a total lack of vitamin C, found in fresh
fruit and green vegetables, is one of the oldest diseases known
to humankind. It was endemic in Northern Europe during the
Middle Ages, particularly in winter when fresh food was
unavailable. One of the biggest killers ever, it is thought to
have killed more men at sea than died in either shipwreck or in
battle. The discovery by the naval doctor James Lind that
citrus fruit (limes and lemons) could prevent and cure scurvy
led to the British being called Limeys.

During the industrial revolution the mass of the population

continued to eat a deficient diet, although more widespread cultivation of the potato (which contains vitamin C) did help. Fresh fruit was not a normal part of town dwellers' diet: it was too expensive, and was not available throughout the year. Scurvy continued to kill, until the production of fresh fruit and vegetables increased, incomes rose, and large quantities of citrus fruit started to be imported.

Nowadays improved transport and refrigeration mean that there should be no problem. Production of fruit in Britain has increased considerably during the twentieth century. But in any one week about a third of British households buy no fresh fruit at all. Millions of Britons spend more money on sweets than on fruit. They do not die from scurvy, but many people are only eating the bare minimum of vitamin C each day. Their health may suffer.

Trifles and Telephones

Why are we not very keen on eating fruit? Quite apart from the fact that fresh fruit does not fit into the structure of most British meals (sugary trifle remains our favourite pudding), there may be another reason.

It is commonly held in Britain that eating too much fruit will have a catastrophic effect on the bowels. One fruit too many and there will be terrible consequences. But what is diarrhoea? As individuals we all know what we mean by abnormal bowel function. The question is, what is normal by international standards?

Research on this delicate subject has found that the typical British adult produces 4 oz of stools per day. In countries where the diet includes large amounts of wholegrain cereals, fruit and vegetables, things are entirely different. The perfect specimen is apparently to be found in rural East Africa, at 5.00 a.m. by the side of the road. It is large, pale and soft, so soft it settles into a circular shape, with a diameter of some 5 to 6 inches. This stool tends to float in water.

Now that surely sounds a bit abnormal? Pale? Round? Soft? 'Normal' in Britain means a sausage shaped item; tending to be dark in appearance, certainly on the hard side compared with the East African variety.

In countries where fresh vegetables, beans, fruit and wholegrain cereals are eaten regularly and in large amounts, daily output is over twice that of the British adult, who produces only five to seven stools per week. By international standards we are abnormal. As a nation we are constipated. We build up libraries in our lavatories to while away the time. The Japanese install telephones in hotel lavatories because they know that Western businessmen need to spend so long there.

What is the effect on health of so constipating a diet? Many intestinal disorders have been linked with lack of dietary fibre, which is found in fruit, vegetables and whole cereals: piles (haemorrhoids), diverticular disease, intestinal polyps (lumps on the inner wall of the colon), appendicitis (almost unknown in countries where the NACNE-type diet is eaten), colon cancer. The links between diet and these and many other illnesses are still being studied. But we know that, at the very least, nearly all constipation could be relieved tomorrow if we ate healthier food. If all of us doubled our consumption of fresh fruit, that would be a good start. Fruit, vegetables and wholegrain cereals all affect the quantity and quality of stools produced. Wholegrain cereal foods have the most potent effect of all the foods so far studied Fruit also produces the right results. Much more of it is needed to help unblock the system and begin the process of lavatorial re-education.

Pip-Pip to the Pitmaston Pine Apple

Fruit provides dietary fibre and also vitamins. The fresher the fruit, the more vitamin C it will contain. Fruit contains various minerals. Fresh fruit is particularly high in potassium, which protects against high blood pressure.

When edible, the skin and seeds (pips) of fruit provide fibre and essential oils.

The nutritional value of fresh fruit is far superior to that of canned fruit. Frozen fruit is usually better than canned, but the vitamin C content falls the longer it is stored.

We have eaten the same 2½ oz of fruit a day for thirty years, but the fruits we eat have changed. A generation ago, fruit meant chiefly apples, oranges and bananas. The variety has widened. Peaches, plums, strawberries, greengages, grapes, tangerines, satsumas and, recently, some more exotic fruits are becoming popular. Fresh mangoes, paw-paws, lychees, guavas, kiwifruit, persimmons all appear more frequently on market stalls and in supermarkets. It is quite likely that the choice will further expand dramatically during the next ten or twenty years, because only a very small proportion of the world's tropical fruits have been grown commercially. The jungles of Latin America still abound with edible fruits unknown to the world at large. New Zealand has taken the initiative in producing exotic fruits in recent years. They launched the kiwifruit, and there are several others in the pipeline.

But what about traditional British fruits? Cox's Orange Pippin, Golden Delicious and Granny Smith have overrun the apple market in recent years. What has happened to the Blenheim, one of Britain's highest prized apples in the nineteenth century? Or James Grieve, or the Pitmaston Pine Apple, or Ashmead's Kernel or the dozens of apple varieties listed in old horticultural journals? New varieties of apple have been introduced in this century, but many more have vanished, dismissed as poor croppers, or because they store badly. Most supermarkets and greengrocers only sell one or two varieties. They do not seem to be interested in stocking new varieties as they come into season. Maybe it is too much trouble.

The incentives for farmers to grow different varieties are not very great. EEC and government subsidies on fruit production are small by comparison with those on dairy, cereal and meat products. Little money is spent on advertising fresh fruit, because it is a low-profit margin commodity with little 'added value'.

Strawberries, another British favourite, are much cheaper and much more widely available in the growing season than they used to be. But the number of commercial varieties grown is very small. Although the physical quality is good, they are tasteless by comparison with the home-grown variety. This is because they are cultivated at maximum speed for maximum yield. Good flavour is usually not a priority. What matters is that they do not get mildew and are red and shiny.

Adieu to Flavour

The appearance of British fruit has undoubtedly changed greatly since the war: when did you last bite into an apple and meet a friendly earwig? And the volume of fruit has increased to keep up with the post-war increase in population. But as with vegetables, production relies on the intensive use of pesticides.

If you see a different shaped or different coloured fruit in your greengrocers, try it. The flavour might be good. The British fruit industry and the EEC seem to believe that the Great British Public wants its fruit uniform in shape and colour; variety of taste is almost immaterial. More to the point might be the fact that supermarkets like their fruit to be all the same size. That way they can sell you six for 50p and the total weight will vary little. They can also pack fruit in trays of uniform size. Uniformity of appearance is often an indication of a bland and boring taste.

The EEC discourages diversity by insisting on strict grading standards – bland uniform bureaucrats go home contented, after insisting on bland uniform fruit. Tiny apples are rejected. But can a child munch its way through a 6 oz apple, let alone keep hold of it? Small apples are ideal for little fingers. It is a very wasteful practice to reject small fruit as sub-standard. Much of it that could be used in fruit juice is destroyed each year.

Dried and Canned Fruit

All dried fruits make good snacks for children who want something sweet. They contain large amounts of dietary fibre and many minerals.

Whole food shops have a much wider choice than most supermarkets. Dried bananas, apples, pineapples, hunzas (like apricots), as well as the more common figs, raisins, sultanas and currants can be bought more cheaply, and in bulk (and often without artificial preservatives).

Canned fruits were introduced when processed sugars and fruit became cheaper in the late nineteenth and early twentieth centuries. Purchases reached a peak in the late 1960s, but have since declined. Just as well, for some contain a lot of sugars. A small can of fruit in heavy syrup may contain more than 8 teaspoons of sugar. A small can in light syrup may contain 5 teaspoons.

Sainsburys were one of the first supermarkets to introduce canned fruits in natural fruit juice. Choose these in preference to sweetened varieties.

Juice – the Real Thing?

Fruit juice is becoming more popular. In the course of 1982 we drank 10 litres each, compared with only 3½ litres in 1978. Orange juice is the sort we like best. It accounts for two thirds of all the fruit juice drunk in Britain.

How good is fruit juice in tins and cartons? It certainly does not contain the same amount of vitamin C as fresh fruit. The level could be anything from 0 per cent to about 60 per cent of the amount in fresh fruit.

The vast majority of these juices are extracted in the country where the fruit is grown, then dehydrated and shipped to Britain, where they are rehydrated and put into cartons. Vitamin C levels deteriorate if the juice is stored a long time in warm conditions. Even under perfect conditions, the amount falls with time.

Not all fruit juices are as pure as they seem. If the product is called orange 'drink' rather than orange 'juice', then it is made with oranges and also with other things such as sugars. Read the labels, and you may find a list of preservatives, sugars, artificial sweeteners, citric acid and so forth, where you expected only to find fruit juice. Appeel Orange, for example, provides you with about two teaspoons of sugar per glass! Better to peel an orange.

Pure fruit juices are 100 per cent better for children than fizzy drinks, squashes and lemonades, but a piece of fresh fruit is better still.

The supermarket shelves are lined with bottles of sweetened drinks. The majority contain absolutely nothing of nutritional value. Their chief ingredient is sugars (although the manufacturers have developed a cunning little habit of telling you the contents of diluted squash, so that water comes first on the list of ingredients, rather than sugars!), followed by colourings, flavourings and preservatives. These drinks are quite useless to anyone but the dentists and the slimming clubs who they help to keep in business.

Even the drinks with a healthy reputation, such as Ribena and Lucozade, are a nutritional disaster*. One glass of Lucozade can contain no less than eight teaspoons of sugars, while a glass of Ribena has five! There are four teaspoons of sugar to every medium-size bottle of tonic water or ginger ale, five for one of bitter lemon. If you must drink these things, choose the artificially sweetened ones instead.

Lastly, beware the drinks that say they are sweetened with glucose or fructose syrup. They are just as bad for you as the ones sweetened with other forms of sugar.

---

*Until 1985 Ribena, together with other blackcurrant 'health drinks', contained amaranth (E123), a coal-tar dye banned in the USA because it can cause adverse reactions, including cancer, in animals. Amaranth is permitted in Britain. In 1985 Beechams, the drug and food firm responsible for the manufacture of Ribena, made it available without amaranth.

EAT FRESH NUTS

Nuts are bulging with nourishment. Most nuts are low in saturated and high in polyunsaturated fats. They also contain dietary fibre, and are crammed with minerals. They are a far healthier snack than sweets or crisps, biscuits and cakes. However, it is not wise to give nuts to toddlers because they can easily choke on them. For older children dried fruit and nuts, or nuts alone, are a good snack between meals.

Buy unsalted peanuts. Roasted peanuts are often cooked with additional oil. The dry-roasted ones are smothered in artificial flavouring and colourings.

Nuts are good in salads. Dry-roasted sesame seeds, cashew nuts, sunflower seeds and almonds (or other seeds) are a delicious addition to many dishes. Nuts tend to be expensive, but you do not need to use very many. Buy them in whole food shops with a high turnover; stale nuts are not worth eating.

Coconut oil is over 80 per cent saturated, by contrast; so avoid coconut sweets and biscuits. Used occasionally in curries, dried coconut is not harmful. But used regularly, it can provide quite a lot of saturated fat.

Fruit and Nuts – A Summary of the Advice

• Eat more fruit of all kinds.

• Eat more fresh fruit salads. Try exotic fruits.

• Prefer whole fruit to fruit juices.

• Avoid 'fruit' squashes and cordials.

• Eat fruit or nuts as snacks rather than confectionery.

CHAPTER 12

Alcohol

A FOOD, OR A DRUG? HEAVY DRINKING AND ALCOHOLISM.
IS THERE A 'SAFE LIMIT'? SHOULD PREGNANT WOMEN DRINK?

This book might have been entitled *The Food and Drink Scandal*; for the record of successive governments on alcohol policy has been, and is, a national disgrace. One major reason, as with cigarette smoking, is money, or rather revenue: in 1985 it was reckoned (by the *British Medical Journal*) that the Exchequer collects £4,000 million a year from tax levied on alcoholic drinks – nearly a quarter of the cost of the NHS.

That is not the end of the story. For some time now the general policy of the Chancellor of the Exchequer at budget time has been to raise the price of cigarettes roughly in line with the retail price index; so that cigarettes, now, cost about the same in real terms as they did thirty years ago. Two Conservative Chancellors (Sir Geoffrey Howe and Nigel Lawson) have referred to cigarette smoking as a public health problem.

Meanwhile, cynics point out, revenue from the tax on cigarettes continues to rise. And while men – middle class men, mainly – are smoking less, women are smoking more. The Royal College of Physicians, in their fourth anti-smoking report, *Smoking or Health*, published in 1984, estimated that smoking causes 100,000 unnecessary deaths in Britain every year.

But the situation with drinking is just as alarming. (In this chapter, 'drinking' means 'drinking alcoholic drinks'.) For in the last thirty years the tax on alcohol has not kept pace with rising prices of other goods. Far from it. In 1980, compared with 1950, in real terms, beer was two thirds the price. Whisky was one quarter the 1950 price in 1980. As a result, according to a survey commissioned by the Consumers' Association and published in the November 1984 edition of *Which?* magazine, in the last twenty years the drinking of beer has increased by one quarter, and the drinking of spirits has doubled. Drinking of wine, further encouraged by EEC agreements, has trebled. Between 1950 and 1976 drunkenness convictions doubled, and deaths from cirrhosis of the liver, caused by alcohol abuse, increased 60 per cent.

Why has alcohol become more and more cheap? After all, as has been discovered with cigarettes the higher the tax the greater the revenue, even when consumption drops.

One reason is that doctors have not yet recognized, as they have with smoking, that drinking is a major public health problem. Indeed, the rate of heavy drinking and alcoholism among doctors (and politicians) is very high, whereas the rate of smoking among doctors is now low. A standard joke about doctors and drinking is the one about a conference on alcohol: "10.00 a.m. – 'The effect of alcohol on the unborn child'. 11.00 – 'Murders: is drunkenness the true cause?'. 11.45 – 'Alcohol and heart disease'. 12.30 – Bar opens."

Certainly, there are no signs, as with smoking, that better educated or better paid people are drinking less. Quite the reverse.

The last Labour government commissioned the Central Policy Review Staff (the now disbanded 'Think Tank') to produce a report, 'Alcohol Policies', which they did, in May 1979, around the time that NACNE was being set up. The Conservative government was elected in June 1979. The report has never been published.

It was suppressed and, unlike the NACNE report, remains suppressed. In April 1982 a leaked copy of the report was published from Sweden, in English, but the attitude of the Department of Health remains that it does not exist. No national newspaper has published its findings, although it was mentioned in *The Times* in 1983, and in *The Observer* on 7 October 1984, in a leading article calling for its publication.

Booze is good for business and for employment. There are around three quarters of a million people in Britain employed in the manufacture, distribution and sale of alcoholic drinks. Exports of drink, notably Scotch whisky, are now worth over £1,000 million a year. Drink is an excellent commodity. It has become easy for young people to buy alcoholic drinks in off-licences and supermarkets (where drink is stocked next to sweets, chocolates and crisps). Around forty MPs, mostly Conservatives, have known interests in the alcohol industry.

Booze is what makes the world go round, in many people's minds. (For others, it makes the world go round and round.) There are issues with drinking that do not apply to smoking. Pubs, wine bars and parties are places and times to be sociable; lunch and dinner are occasions for business, also. A non-smoker is no longer at a social disadvantage (indeed, nowadays there is pressure against smokers). But most people find it hard not to drink on social occasions. Teetotallers are regarded with some suspicion (killjoy? reformed drunk?). And whatever the advertisements for Marlboro cigarettes may suggest, nobody would regard smoking two packs of cigarettes in an evening as a test of manhood, whereas getting legless is a popular hobby for many men, as is boasting about getting legless, before and after the event. Drunks are figures of fun to comedians. Falling into the canal after closing time is the stuff of myth in the North (as recorded in the Andy Capp cartoon strip).

On a more sophisticated level, drink is celebrated as one of the pleasures of civilization. Newspapers employ wine correspondents. Wine books and magazines are published so that you can learn what is what and when was when. The

Campaign for Real Ale has given downmarket drinking some chic. Champagne is kept on ice in the bath, or popped, or smashed, to launch weddings, infants, or liners. And most people would find a substantial meal, certainly if eaten out, incomplete without wine and/or other drink. Alcohol weaves through our culture (as do alcoholics).

A Food, or a Drug?

Alcoholic drinks are considered as food, in the sense that they can be consumed as part of a meal; that they taste good and their taste is considered to be part of the experience of a meal; that some alcoholic drinks contain some nourishment; and that alcohol contributes to total calorie consumption.

The NACNE report concentrated on this last point, stating that, as a national average, 6 per cent of calories consumed are in the form of alcohol, and that within the UK the range is substantial, from an average of 4 per cent in London and southeast England, to 9 per cent in Scotland. In terms of actual drink, 6 per cent of calories on a daily basis is very roughly a pint of beer or cider, two glasses of wine or sherry, or a double of spirits.

Seen as food, sugar and confectionery is a fair analogy for alcohol and drinks. Like sugars, alcohol itself supplies no nourishment, only calories (and considerably more, per unit of weight, than sugars do). Like confectionery, alcoholic drinks may contain nourishment: there are small quantities of some vitamins in beer, and both wine and beer contain minerals, for instance (nothing of value in spirits). But do not fool yourself into thinking that alcoholic drinks are nourishing, or a 'tonic', or anything of that sort. A drink may cheer you up, but that's not the nourishment in it working, that's the alcohol.

So the more alcohol you drink, the less room you will have for nourishing food: the same point applies here as to sugars, saturated fats and highly processed starches.

But is there any harm in drinking modestly – say, a couple of drinks a day? (One 'drink' is defined as a half-pint of beer, a glass of wine, or a single of spirits, all of average strength.) For here, too, most people would see a difference between smoking and drinking; the common view is that smoking is always bad, and the message is Stop; but that modest drinking is all right, and the message is 'a little of what you fancy does you good'. Is this true?

There is still argument between scientists on this point (before and after opening time). But the only really worthwhile discussion, is about whether or not alcohol to some extent protects against heart disease: two subjects of special interest to middle-aged men, which is after all what most leading scientists are.

Some research seems to show that alcohol does indeed have an effect on the blood which should reduce the risk of a heart attack: it increases the proportion of high density lipoprotein, the type of blood fat – bound up with protein – that protects against heart disease; and it in effect makes the blood thinner and so less sticky. Researchers who think that alcohol may to some extent protect against heart disease stress that they are talking about small amounts – back to the 'two drinks a day and no more' recommendation.

The counter argument is, first, that the type of high density lipoprotein increased by alcohol is probably not, as it turns out, helpful. Second, even if alcohol in small quantities does the blood some good, it certainly is no good for the cardiovascular system in general. Third, susceptible people are liable to develop disorders of digestion, the nervous system and the immune system, as a result of fairly modest amounts of alcohol, well before there is any question of serious liver damage. Fourth, women are much more susceptible than men to damage from alcohol, for reasons that are not fully understood, not just to do with being smaller and lighter.

And fifth, alcohol is a drug of addiction, and it is dangerous to think of it as having a pharmaceutical use. It is true that doctors prescribe many drugs whose adverse effects are liable to be at least as damaging as alcohol, but two poisons do not make an elixir.

Heavy Drinking and Alcoholism

The popular image of an alcoholic is of a human wreck sitting in rags and filth on a park bench, propped by a bottle of cider laced with meths. Such people are as untypical of alcoholics, as the teenager found dead in a public lavatory with a needle in his arm is of drug addicts.

How many alcoholics – people suffering from alcohol abuse – are there in Britain? The brewers say 75,000. The Think Tank report, 'Alcohol Policies', says over 500,000. The *British Medical Journal* estimates that the cost of alcohol abuse to industry, together with legal, police and medical costs, was £1,600 million in 1983. A third of all drivers killed in car crashes are drunk. A quarter of all pedestrians killed on the road are killed by drunk drivers. A majority of murders are committed when the murderer is drunk. 'Alcohol Policies' stated of alcohol abuse: 'The trends in misuse justify government concern. Without government initiatives and a better concerted set of policies these trends are likely to continue.'

Sounds familiar, doesn't it?

Most alcoholics are living with their families, doing a job (perhaps with absences on Mondays), driving cars, operating machinery, and not identified as alcoholics. It usually takes some disaster to happen, for the question to be asked. 'Fun loving' people in public life, when interviewed, tend to explain that they are not alcoholics, perhaps meaning that they haven't yet learned to drink while asleep. 'Responsible' people in public life, in court after wrecking property or citizens with their cars when drunk, are reported to have been suffering stress and strain. Magistrates seem sometimes to be understanding when the person in the dock is a magistrate or such-like, unless a policeman has been damaged.

Are you an alcoholic? As a rule of thumb, if you have reached the stage of asking the question, the answer is likely to be yes. There are lots of books with questionnaires on this subject, which range from 'do you sometimes fancy one before opening time?' (a bit dodgy) to 'have you ever woken up with no idea who was in bed with you?' (definitely dodgy).

The NACNE report uses another report, by the Royal College of Psychiatrists, which provides another rule of thumb, about quantity. This suggests that generally speaking anybody who regularly drinks more than four pints of beer, or a bottle of wine, or four doubles of spirits a day, is in danger of becoming alcoholic. This is a very rough and ready guide. Women can tolerate maybe half the amount of alcohol that men can.

As a food, four pints of beer a day, or a bottle of wine, amounts to 20-30 per cent of total energy, for a sedentary person, and makes alcohol bad news, just like sugars. As a drug, regular drinking at this level is dangerous. And from the medical and public health point of view, heavy, including 'regular social', drinking is liable to destroy your liver, in time. The heaviest drinkers in Europe are the French. The biggest public health problem in France is liver disease.

Is There a 'Safe' Limit?

Alcohol is no good for your health, as everybody who has ever asked 'what's your poison?' knows. But heavy drinking is the principal problem. If you are a man and, over a week, you average one to two drinks a day, that's all right. If you are a woman and, over a week, you average less than a drink a day, that's all right too – with one vital exception – see below. Savour the quality of a glass of real ale, or fine wine, or malt whisky, or vintage champagne, or whatever makes your taste-buds race; but, for the rest, become a connoisseur of mineral water.

Should Pregnant Women Drink?

Absolutely not. One of the most carefully guarded secrets about alcohol, is that it is a teratogen. 'Teratogen' means 'creator of monsters': a teratogen is a poison that is liable, if taken in pregnancy, to result in deformed or retarded babies. The drug thalidomide, for example, is a teratogen. So is nuclear fall-out.

If a woman is starved of nourishment her periods are liable to stop: this is nature's way of protecting her against a pregnancy her body could not sustain. If a woman is semi-starved of nourishment she may become pregnant but the foetus is liable to abort: this is the natural protection of the unborn child who, if born, would be liable to be damaged.

But if a woman is erratically nourished and becomes pregnant, the natural processes in her body are liable, effectively, to become confused. In Britain women are well-nourished in the sense of eating every day, and eating some healthy food most if not all days. This encourages the body to tolerate pregnancy. This is why drinking alcohol (together with other drugs, like the Pill and antibiotics, and junk food) is dangerous: for there is a real risk of a baby that will turn out to be if not obviously damaged, then frankly, rather stupid. To put it another way, the children of mothers who drink are at risk of not reaching their full potential.

The children of mothers who drink heavily, are at risk of the 'foetal alcohol syndrome'. This stigma is not as severe as Downs Syndrome (mongolism). 'FAS' children have rather stubby noses and a correspondingly long upper lip. Such children are liable to suffer physical and mental retardation. In America the Surgeon General has stated that, for the sake of their babies, women who are pregnant or who are considering pregnancy should not drink. A study reported in the *British Medical Journal* in 1983 concluded 'a policy of total abstinence from alcohol from before conception if possible and certainly during pregnancy, appears to be the only sensible way to ensure an unaffected child with full intellectual potential'.

The Future

'Alcohol Policies' recommended no change in the licensing laws, saying that the government 'should not lightly run the risks that longer hours are likely to bring'. In 1985 the Conservative government was being encouraged by the brewers and distillers to 'liberalize' the licensing hours in the name of freedom, and allow pubs to open at all hours.

Alcohol – A Summary of the Advice

- For health, don't drink.
- For safety, keep below two drinks a day (men) and one drink a day (women).
- To avoid alcoholism, keep below four pints of beer or a bottle of wine a day (men) and half this amount (women).
- Women who are thinking of having a baby should drink no alcohol before conception and throughout pregnancy.

CHAPTER 13

Babies and Toddlers

ADDITIVES, ALLERGY AND BEHAVIOUR PROBLEMS.
BREAST IS BEST.
DEXTROSE, GLUCOSE, AND ALL THE LITTLE '-OSE'S.
TODDLERS' MILK: TRUTH IS AN OFFICIAL SECRET.

The food industry knows that parents, and mothers in particular, worry about the food they give their small children. That is why the number of different baby foods on our shop shelves is growing. But how good are they? And how necessary is it to give a baby 'special' food? What is the best you can do for your child?

Additives, Allergy and Behaviour Problems

In 1984, a growing number of mothers learned about the effects of food additives on children's behaviour. Many newspapers carried 'amazing stories' of unmanageable, demonic, hyperactive children transformed into normal, well behaved little darlings after a change to a whole food diet and, in particular, avoidance of sugars and artificial colourings and other additives in processed foods.

It was the mothers who had taken things into their own hands, following research findings in the USA that linked processed foods with hyperactivity and unruly behaviour. This research has been largely ignored by British doctors, with the exception of a handful who are interested in allergy and all its manifestations, be it migraine, spots, bad temper, or sleeplessness.

How much evidence is there that these things are caused by food? Research on this subject is difficult to conduct in an unbiased manner, but the carefully conducted studies done to date certainly show that some children (and adults too) are very sensitive to certain additives and contaminants in foods. The artificial colour tartrazine (E102) is perhaps the best known, but there are others.

The foods that contain these things tend in any case to be heavily processed, to consist largely of processed fats, added sugars, processed starches, as well as additives. In short, they generally tend to be foods of poor nutritional value which are in any case best avoided.

What should your child eat to start life in the healthiest way?

Breast is Best

Breast milk is unquestionably of superior nutritional quality to any of the artificial varieties. It contains anti-infective agents which protect the baby; it contains just the right amount of protein. And, provided the mother herself eats healthy food, the fatty acid composition of human milk is ideal. Vegan and vegetarian mothers in the UK have more of the essential polyunsaturates in their milk than do 'carnivorous' mothers.

Breast feeding on demand will satisfy most infants for at least three months; a small baby tends to need less extra food at an older age than a large one, but of course it will depend on the amount of milk produced.

The best advice for any pregnant woman is to make sure the hospital knows you want to breast feed right from the start. Do not allow the nurses to give your baby sugar-water on the first day, because human colostrum is far healthier. Infants allowed to breast feed on demand from within minutes of the birth establish a more contented feeding schedule than those that have been 'interfered' with.

Dextrose, Glucose and All the Little '-ose's

At some time after 3 months, extra food is necessary. What should it be? For a start avoid all foods containing added salt, added sugars, artificial colours and preservatives. Choose foods which are low in saturated fats. Healthy infant food is really no different from healthy adult food, but it will of course need to be prepared so the baby can eat it.

Some of the baby food manufacturers are rather keen on sugars. Take a look at the list of ingredients of special baby foods and what do you find? Dextrose, glucose, fructose, and others. In an attempt to recapture the health-conscious mother's attention, 'low sugar' or 'reduced sugar' babyfoods have recently appeared. But beware; many of them have almost as much sugar as before – the only difference is that sugars are added as glucose (or dextrose) rather than sucrose. And special baby foods are also expensive, even though they may save time. Some of these special foods are of good nutritional quality, but you will need to check the list of contents carefully.

Protein: Not a Problem

A healthy baby with a good appetite will get all the protein he or she needs from the type of food recommended in this book. Plant proteins are just as good as those from animal foods, provided the foods are varied.

Toddlers' Milk: Truth Is an Official Secret

Here, there has been some confusion and controversy. When the Department of Health COMA sub-committee published its report *Diet and Cardiovascular Disease* in 1984, the recommendations it made were *for the nation as a whole*: less fats, less saturated fats in particular, perhaps a little more polyunsaturated fats, less salt. The report went on to suggest how industry, the government, doctors and health educationists might achieve the changes for the nation as a whole. However, after the committee had finished their deliberations, an addition was made. This is what it said:

> The recommendations that follow are intended mainly for older children and for young and middle-aged adults; . . . They are not intended for infants (i.e. those under one year of age) and the recommendation for fat is not appropriate for children under the age of five. The advice relating to infants and young children . . . is from the Panel on Child Nutrition of the Committee on Medical Aspects of Food Policy.

What had happened is that the COMA Cardiovascular sub-committee considered that everybody, including young children, would benefit from eating less fatty foods. Atherosclerosis starts in early childhood, therefore it is logical to prevent it from infancy onwards. But the COMA sub-committee on child nutrition banged the table and said British children must have their full-fat milk. There was no scientific debate, no evidence was presented to show that milk fat is essential for children, and the Panel on Child Nutrition wrote into the report 'This recommendation [to reduce fats, and particularly saturated fats] is not intended for infants; or for children below the age of five who usually obtain a substantial proportion of dietary energy from cow's milk.' When questioned about this, a member of the COMA Child Nutrition sub-committee replied, 'I've signed the Official Secrets Act; I cannot comment.'

Health visitors, who advise mothers about infant feeding, are confused. Their nutrition training is minimal; they know little about the development of heart disease. They 'believe in' milk, because that is what they have been taught. What should you do if you have a baby?

First, consider the fact that babies around the world move gradually from mother's milk, which they drink for many months more than the average British baby, on to adult foods. For most societies around the world, milk is, at most, a very minor item in an adult's diet. Even the Masai tribe in East Africa, of whom the proponents of dairy foods are so fond, eat much less saturated fat than we do because after drinking about the same amount of milk as we do (some 4 pints per person per week) they do not eat any saturated fats from cakes, biscuits, sweets, artificially hardened fats and so on. Their diet is very frugal. (And the blood they drink is very rich in essential polyunsaturated fats.) So the net result is that despite drinking milk, and eating lean meat, their saturated fats consumption is low.

Second, most dietitians, nutritionists, doctors, health visitors and nurses have a strong emotional (as opposed to scientific) attachment to full-fat milk, which has its roots in early twentieth-century medicine and research and in the years of poverty during the industrial revolution and beyond. Had those same early researchers been aware of the effects of large amounts of saturated dairy fats on the blood circulation, their advice would have been very different.

Third, there are many children who cannot drink milk because they have a deficiency of a digestive enzyme in their intestines which leads to diarrhoea and even vomiting when the child drinks milk (called lactose intolerance). These children grow perfectly well without milk, provided they are given a healthy mixed diet. And here is the crux of the matter. Growing children, like the rest of us, need good quality food: fresh fruit and vegetables, wholemeal bread, fish, lean meat, beans, essential polyunsaturated fats. What they do not need is refined sugars, saturated fats, refined flour, artificial flavours, colours and preservatives.

The difficulty is that for many children in Britain today, particularly the poor, milk is about the best food they get, even with its saturated fats. For the poorest children eat the least fresh food, and the most processed sugars, fats and starches. For them the minerals and vitamins of milk are more important, but only because the rest of their diet is of such poor quality. So the answer to mothers of young children is: wean your babies on to healthy food. If the baby is hungry, keep feeding it! Do not worry about overweight in a toddler unless he or she eats a lot of sugars or fatty foods. Good quality oils can be used for cooking, and will boost the energy content of meals for a small child with a small appetite in a much healthier way than added sugars and dairy fats. If you want your child to drink a lot of milk, try semi-skimmed instead of full-fat milk. The Canadians and Americans have been feeding their children on it for years with no ill-effects so far recorded. This advice is against that of the DHSS COMA Panel on Child Nutrition, and the authors of this book make no apology for it. The valuable nutrients of milk are in the watery part, the skim: this is where all the important vitamins, minerals and protein are to be found.

One word of warning: babies of under six months should never be given ordinary cow's milk whether full-fat, semi-skilled or completely skimmed. The reason is that it is designed for calves, and the human kidney is unhappy when confronted with a load of high sodium, high protein, cow's milk. That is why tins of milk powder are labelled 'Not suitable for babies', and why baby milk powders have to be especially modified to ensure that the mineral and protein content is safe for the human infant. So never give babies doorstep milk; try to breast feed for as long as possible, and wean on to healthy foods. Your baby will thank you in later life.

Babies and Toddlers – A Summary of the Advice

- Breast feed on demand for as long as possible, or at least 3 months.

- Avoid sugary, salty foods high in saturated fats.

- Avoid additives.

- Never give 'doorstep' cow's milk to a child of under 6 months.

- Semi-skimmed milk is a healthy alternative to full milk for toddlers eating a varied diet.

CHAPTER 14

Slimming and Exercise

DIETS DO NOT WORK. HIGH IN NOURISHMENT, LOW IN CALORIES.
HOW TO KEEP CHILDREN SLIM.
LOSING FAT AND GAINING HEALTH.

At a rough guess, about half the people who read this book want to lose weight. Are you one of them? Trying – and, usually, failing – to solve the problem of overweight is an obsessional pastime in Britain. About two thirds of adult women and one third of adult men are thinking of slimming at any one time. Few people with a weight problem have not tried at least one of the diets constantly published in books, magazines and newspapers. Most have tried not one but several.

Women's magazines and publishers know how desperate their readers can be. Grapefruit diets one month, steak diets the next, followed by fruit fasts, fibre plans and, latest of all, the diet that actually encourages you to eat sweets between meals. The Liquorice All-sorts diet was featured in the *Daily Mail* in 1984. The motivation to slim for most people is not primarily to be healthy, but to look better.

The effects of overweight on health are not immediately apparent. Like most common health problems in Britain, overweight develops slowly and is more obvious in adulthood.

It is associated with heart disease, high blood pressure, gall bladder disease, diabetes, respiratory disorders, arthritis and a generally unfit physical condition. And it is not only severe obesity that causes illness. Even mild overweight is strongly linked with early illness and death. But most people do not make the connection between their superfluous fat and the threat of ill-health.

With about one third of the adult population of Britain overweight, and still more of us overfat (apparently the right weight for our height, but with handfuls of fat tissue where lean tissue should be), the nation has a problem. How can we turn ourselves from fat and flabby to lean and healthy? Will the diet books help? What about exercise?

As a nation we not only eat badly, we are unfit. The human body is not designed to travel everywhere – or most places – by means of the internal combustion engine, any more than it is designed to consume foods high in calories and low in nourishment (such as fats, sugars, and alcohol). The human frame is designed for regular exercise using two large muscle groups, the legs and the arms. This type of exercise is called walking. We should do more of it.

But if we are overweight, or overfat, isn't dieting the only way to slim?

DIETS DO NOT WORK

The diets advocated for weight loss, whether dished out by the hospital dietitian or the station bookstall, have one thing in common. All end up by recommending a reduced calorie intake. In other words, if the average energy (calorie) expenditure in a day is about 2,000 to 2,300 for women, diets of 1,000 to 1,500 calories should produce weight loss. The diets differ in the type of food they recommend: fat, fibre, fruit, low carbohydrate, high carbohydrate, meat, have been recommended. A Mars Bar diet was once commissioned from the University of Surrey, by industry. The most sensible of these diets are likely to come from the hospital dietitians who have no vested interests or nutritional obsessions, the silliest from individuals who advocate single-food diets, and the most dangerous from those who advocate very low calorie diets (around 300 calories a day) and powdered diets in tins.

But do they work in the long term? The experience of most dieters is that they do not. Initial weight loss is rapid, then slows down a bit, then stops. If target weight is reached, and only a minority of dieters achieve this, it is only sustained by a few. Most overweight people feel that they face a life-long battle against the bulge. To win it, they are to be for ever deprived of the fattening foods the rest of the population continues to eat at will. They are encouraged to believe that failure at dieting is caused by greed combined with the wrong kind of metabolism.

The arguments against low-calorie diet regimes are more extensively dealt with by Geoffrey Cannon and Hetty Einzig in their book *Dieting Makes You Fat* and will not be discussed in any detail here. The suggested programme outlined below for treating overweight does not rely on counting calories – or indeed on counting anything. It does not turn eating into an arithmetic minefield. It is not designed for instant spectacular weight loss, nor even for a few weeks' shedding of pounds. It is a plan for lifelong healthy eating. It is, in fact, identical to the plan suggested in the NACNE report for the population at large, in other words, food low in fats, processed sugars and alcohol, and high in fibre. There is no magic ingredient for weight loss.

High in Nourishment, Low in Calories

Follow the advice in the rest of this book and you will be well on the way to reducing your body fat. Energy-heavy foods are those that contain a lot of fat, processed sugars and alcohol. Most of us by now know what they are: cakes, biscuits, sweetened drinks, pies, sausages, chips, fried foods, most cheeses, cream, butter, margarine, cooking fats, fat on milk, meat fat, sweets, ice cream, sweetened breakfast cereals, alcoholic drinks. If you have read the rest of this book, the list will be very familiar. Most of these foods should be eaten only sparingly.

Fatness is caused by eating foods heavy in calories and poor in essential nutrients. Whole foods – cereals, vegetables and fruit – are not only rich in nourishment, but also contain few calories for their bulk. Bulky food is satisfying. If you think that bread and potatoes are fattening, you will be interested to know that two scientific experiments have shown that people who eat vast quantities of bread or potatoes tend to lose weight. They do not have room to consume too many calories.

People are confused about what is good food for slimming and what is bad food, largely because of the nonsenses preached by diet books. What about the 'common sense' advice that the way to slim is to cut down on all the food you eat? This advice is wrong, too. Don't be in any doubt about it: the foods to avoid are fat, sugars and alcohol. The advice is very specific.

Food for the slightly overweight (up to a stone overweight) is no different from food for the slim. It should include a lot of bulky cereals and vegetables, such as potatoes, rice, pasta, noodles and bread, and a lot of fresh fruit, beans and vegetables. It should be particularly low in fats, sugars and alcohol. That way the food will contain essential nutrients such as minerals, vitamins and protein, but few empty calories.

People with a more serious weight problem (well over a stone overweight) should cut fats, sugars and alcohol right out, drink skimmed milk, eat only low-fat cheeses (cottage, Quark, curd, ricotta, but check the fat level), avoid all cakes and biscuits, pies and sausages. Eat poultry and fish in preference to red meats. And eat bread, potatoes and other cereals together with beans, fresh fruit and vegetables to fill you up. Remember that starchy carbohydrate foods are not fattening unless you cook or eat them with fat and sugars. To make sure you get enough essential fats, have three teaspoons of an oil which is high in polyunsaturates every day.

For the seriously obese (for example, a woman of average height weighing 15 stone or more) the advice is not so simple. The vast majority of overweight people are not more than a few pounds or stones overweight. Those with a very serious weight problem are likely to need expert advice. If you are in this position, ask your GP to refer you to a qualified dietitian who can offer help and support. Remember that doctors are not trained in nutrition. Most GPs know less about dieting and nutrition than their overweight patients, so you may have to put up with discouraging remarks, exhortations to find a bit more will power, sort out your psychological problems, etc.

A small minority of the population is prone to severe obesity, just as a small minority is prone to develop extremely high blood pressure or blood cholesterol. In actual numbers, this group of individuals is very small. The main problem is the far, far greater number of people with slight or moderate but harmful overweight; just as there is a far greater number of individuals with harmful moderately raised blood cholesterol. The difference with severe obesity is that it is only too visible. The slimmer majority greatly underestimates the misery caused by severe obesity.

How to Keep Children Slim

An overweight child is more likely to become an overweight adult. These children are seen rather frequently in Britain. Stand outside a school gate and watch them going in and out. Watch them also trotting along to the local sweet and chip shops for their lunch or late afternoon snack.

Overweight and obese children are handicapped in sports, and they are more likely to be unpopular with their classmates. They are being prevented from leading fulfilling lives from an early age.

If your child is overweight, or over-fat, be very particular about the food he or she eats. Children have one advantage over adults when it comes to weight loss: growth. Growth is fuelled by food and body fat. If you switch to a healthy diet, high in essential nutrients but low in empty calories, you will encourage a fat child to grow into a slim adult.

Do not deprive an overweight child of filling bread and potatoes. Give him or her sandwiches in preference to sweets and chips. Ask at school why full-cream milk is given to the children, and why the school dinners have such a high proportion of fatty, sweet foods to choose from. Ask why nutrition is not taught as a routine to primary and secondary school children. And if your child learns cookery at school, what sort of dishes are prepared? Are they healthy? Or are they meals for constipation and a heart attack later in life?

Children sometimes do not like taking advice from their parents. If you have a seriously overweight child, ask the school sports department, the local authority sports centre and the community dietitian (who can be contacted via the dietetics department at your local hospital) if they can provide a special class for overweight children at which both healthy nutrition and sports are taught in an entertaining way. These services are provided for the benefit of the whole community.

EXERCISE: KEEP IT UP

If you are overweight, dieting by itself is not the answer. It is unhealthy and, usually, futile to go on a very strict diet regime. Regular exercise will help to build up your muscles and speed up metabolic rate. It should be an integral part of your weight loss programme.

What sort of exercise should you do?

If you are very overweight, then it would be foolish to dash outside and run half a mile. Overweight can strain the joints, so the best sort of exercise is one where your weight is supported. Swimming is excellent exercise. Or try cycling, but gently at first. Or just walking. Start by walking briskly, and increase the length of the walk gradually. Do it regularly, four times a week.

Weight loss through healthy eating and exercise will only happen gradually, so don't expect the fat to fall off overnight. It may take three to six months to tone up your muscles sufficiently to have much effect on your metabolic rate. And once the weight is off you will need to keep up the exercise to make sure it stays off.

The 'Aerobic' Vogue

Nowadays a large number of people are talking about formalized 'aerobic' exercise, and it is very much in vogue. What 'aerobic' exercise simply means is activity – brisk walking, jogging, running, swimming, cycling, for instance – that can be maintained at a steady, vigorous pace for at least ten minutes at a time. It includes dance/exercise and also 'aerobics'. Aerobics is now very popular among women, and is good if the trainer is experienced and keeps each exercise session going for ten minutes or so at a time.

Any able-bodied person of any age – certainly anyone aged sixty or under – can undertake regular vigorous activity of this kind. It is a question of finding out what you are capable of, and exercising to just short of the point at which you get out of breath. It is now known that exercising four times a week ('one day on, one day off') for a total of two hours shared between the four sessions, promotes well-being and a general sense of good health, and diminishes the risk of Western diseases, including heart disease, high blood pressure, diabetes, arthritis, brittle bones and depression, as well as overweight. It is vital for people to continue to take exercise throughout their life. Any able-bodied person under sixty who feels up to it need not consult a doctor before undertaking a carefully graduated exercise programme.

Together with good food, exercise promotes health and

well-being. The 1983 report on obesity published by the Royal College of Physicians looked at the decline in physical exercise that has occurred in this century. It concludes that 'too little attention has been paid to the value, on a community basis, of increasing energy expenditure at all ages.' In other words, regular vigorous exercise is vital.

How to Speed Yourself Up

We now know that aerobic exercise speeds up the rate at which the body uses energy – the term for this is the body's 'metabolic rate' – not only as you exercise, but also for some time afterwards. This means that anyone who takes regular vigorous exercise every other day will use more energy at all times, even during sleep. How many extra calories are consumed will vary greatly, depending on the type and intensity of the exercise and on each individual's make-up. Before car ownership became widespread, adults used 450-750 calories a day more on average than we do today. If you make a point of walking, and also sustain a two-hours-a-week exercise programme, you should be able to eat maybe 500 calories a day more, and also lose fat at the same time. You do not have to become a fitness fanatic.

Long-term exercise is the most effective way of losing fat and maintaining weight. Some points to emphasize are the following:

- Exercise must be the right type of exercise, in other words, sustained activity like walking, running or swimming rather than the odd spell of weight-lifting.

- Do not expect remarkable changes during the first three to six months. The body takes time to get used to exercise and to 'tune up'.

- It makes sense to concentrate on losing fat as distinct from losing weight. The great thing is to keep up the exercise for half an hour and more.

Losing Fat and Gaining Health

Many people, especially women, are overfat without being overweight. If, by exercising, you convert 10 lb fat into 10 lb lean tissue, you will look very different, and you will be noticeably slimmer.

Lean tissue weighs more than fat. Regular physical activity will increase the amount of lean tissue in your body, and you will become less flabby. You may not lose weight, but you will lose fat. Lean tissue has a higher metabolic rate than fat tissue. In other words, it uses up more energy and generally ticks over at a faster pace. Exercise to increase the amount of lean tissue in the body will also increase the overall metabolic rate, with subsequent loss of body fat. Specialists in obesity have recently become very interested in this new way of changing the body's shape and composition, as opposed to strict calorie-counted diets. There is also increasing interest among scientists in the value of exercise as a promoter of good health in general.

A Way of Lively Life

Meanwhile, there is no good reason why the rest of us should sit still. Contact your local authority sports centre and find out what sports are available. Ask at your place of work if facilities can be provided (as they are in North America) for sports at lunchtime.

Slimming and Exercise – A Summary of the Advice

- Avoid all added sugars.

- Avoid all saturated fats.

- Eat only very lean meats or preferably fish.

- Eat plenty of fresh fruit, vegetables, beans, whole grain cereals.

- Take regular exercise for four days a week, for a total of two hours.

- 'Endurance'-type exercise is best for fat loss: swimming, running, walking.

Conclusion

LABOUR PLAYS THE HEALTH CARD.
MRS THATCHER AND MR WHIPPY.
WHAT FREEDOM OF CHOICE?
EATING WELL FOR THE REST OF YOUR LIFE.

On 5 March 1985 the Labour Party announced 'The Labour Party – Food Policy a Priority'. At the press conference, Labour front bench spokesman Dr Jeremy Bray denounced the Conservative government policies on food and health as 'chaotic, pointless, perverse and out of date.'

Harking back to the 1960s and the days of Thatcher the Milk Snatcher, health spokesman Frank Dobson added 'the government has abandoned nutritional standards for school meals. This represents a massive impoverishment of children.'

'The Common Agricultural Policy is a direct subsidy of ill-health in Britain,' said Labour Member of the European Parliament Janie Buchan, adding that early signs of heart disease had been detected in Scottish children aged 10.

Labour Plays the Health Card

The Labour Party policy document, for which Dr Bray had special responsibility, followed the lines of the NACNE report. Professor Philip James, together with Sir Richard Doll and Dr Walter Bodmer, were Labour Party advisors. And, happily for the future health prospects of the nation, it turned out that Dr Hugh Trowell, the man who after 30 years as a doctor in Africa had created the original concept of 'Western' diseases, was Dr Bray's father-in-law, and another advisor.

Thus Labour became the first political party capable of forming a government to endorse the NACNE report and its messages.

The Labour policy document called for new food regulations to protect the quality of food by law; new nutritional standards and goals for hospitals and schools; new codes to cut out fraudulent and misleading food advertising; more resources for preventive medicine and health education; policies to make healthy food freely available to poor people; and an all-department government review to achieve policy unity.

Mr Dobson pointed out that 'the system of food pricing isn't natural at all. There's intervention and manipulation now, in favour of unhealthy food. We want sensible intervention.'

As the *Guardian* said in an editorial, the fat was now in the political fire in Britain.

Mrs Thatcher and Mr Whippy

Food and health is not, however, a party political issue; and plenty of Conservative MPs had been thinking about their own health and that of their constituents, ever since the NACNE report became a topic of hot national debate in 1983.

'The food industry knows that the writing is on the wall,' said junior health minister John Patten, interviewed on 4 April 1984. 'One of the jobs of government is to give a big puff of wind to social change that is already happening,' said Mr Patten, and 'it is pretty prudent to reduce the intake of fats, especially saturated fats, in the diet. The marketing opportunities for industry and farming are enormous.'

In Parliament on 16 July 1984, Mr Patten made it clear that the government line was to allow more informed choice of food by finding ways and means to make food labelling more explicit. Taking up a point already made by the authors of this book, published the previous month, Mr Patten referred to:

> the right of the consumer to know as much about the fat content of a packet of sausages as is already known about the contents of a pair of stockings.

Patten agreed that 'when I look at lists of food contents I find it hard to relate them to anything that I understand'. In matters of food and health it is somewhat of a toss-up whether the government department responsible is the Department of Health, or the Ministry of Agriculture, Fisheries and Food. Indeed, problems of food and health that have in the past proved troublesome have tended to be passed from one ministry to the other. However, MAFF minister Michael Jopling reminded the world in 1984 that he was, indeed, Minister of Food, and would be making changes in the labelling of foods, following the publication of the COMA report, *Diet and Cardiovascular Disease*, in June 1984.

Mrs Thatcher is not only a scientist; she is by training a food scientist, who in her early professional life specialized in fat extension, and had the job of putting the 'Whippy' into Mr Whippy ice cream. So in 1984 Britain had a prime minister who knew how to read a food label; and Conservative MPs had reason to believe that she was taking a personal interest in food and health. Mr Jopling was under some pressure to produce results.

This he did, on 12 March 1985. He announced in Parliament that food labels would in due course, by law, carry details of the saturated fat, as well as fat, content of the product when it contributed significantly to fat in the diet. He also announced adjustments to the animal carcass grading system, designed to encourage breeders away from bringing very fatty animals to market. Charles Cockbill, the senior civil servant responsible for the new labelling initiative in MAFF, had already told his colleagues in the EEC that Britain was seeking somewhat more explicit labelling of fats content of foods than was allowed for in

EEC regulations, because of the uniquely high rates of death, and premature death, from heart disease in Britain.

What about sugars? In 1985 government had no plans to introduce food labels with details of sugars content. Curiously, no government has ever commissioned an expert COMA report on sugars and health; not even on the established area of sugars, obesity and tooth decay. Without any such report government makes no moves. This will please the Sugar Bureau, whose director-general, Michael Shersby MP, is also chairman of the Conservative parliamentary party back-bench committee on food and drink.

In 1984 the Sugar Bureau, and its sponsors British Sugar and Tate & Lyle (who between them *are* the British sugar industry) announced a £2 million campaign to promote sugar and protect its record profits.

A deadline was set for all food manufacturers to declare details of all additives in their products (with exceptions), using the European 'E' number system: 1 January 1986. Consumers were becoming particularly interested in additives. A Gallup Poll conducted for Tesco in September 1984 revealed that the biggest health concern among housewives of all social classes, was additives, and cancer. As 1986 approached, some manufacturers, not wanting to give the impression they were selling chemistry sets rather than food, reformulated their products, and advertised them as free of additives. Health had become a selling message.

Conservative policy, as summarized by Ms Mary Coales of MAFF in February 1985, remained 'to move away from compositional standards, to more information on food labels'. The trouble with this policy, which superficially suggests that both industry and consumers should be more free, is that it allows manufacturers to put whatever is good for business into their products, as long as they own up in the small print. Critics feared that abandonment of compositional standards could only lead to the legalized further debasement of food. If all the sausages, biscuits and cakes on the market, apart from those sold at premium prices, contain more and more saturated fats, where is the choice?

What Freedom of Choice?

It is likely that the quality of the food supply in Britain will continue to deteriorate. In January 1985 *The Sunday Times*, in a major feature telling the success story of the Cadbury-Schweppes Wispa bar, estimated that in 1984 total sales of bread in Britain were £1.5 million; of confectionery, £2.5 billion. In 1983 the food industry spent £425 million on advertising, of which sugar, chocolate and confectionery alone accounted for £91.8 million.

The food that is and will remain best for business, in general, is food made by a relatively small number of big, efficiently-run firms, whose operation is highly capital-intensive, and whose highly processed food is packed with 'added value'. This imperative fact of the market will continue to operate under any government, whatever its politics.

If everybody demanded good food and refused inferior alternatives, then of course the industry would make more good food. People in the industry say that the British housewife knows and cares little about food, and is interested only in cheapness and convenience. This story of course suits a capital-intensive industry, geared to produce massive quantities of a small number of lines, which may be given a spurious look of 'variety' by use of artificial flavourings and colourings.

The interests of the British housewife have not been served in this country by the active, informed and campaigning consumer groups of the type that exist in North America, Europe and Australia. In Britain, the Consumers' Association has in part become part of the behind-closed-doors decision-making process, controlled by government, industry and scientific advisors. Indeed, CA and its magazine *Which?* has, certainly in recent years, had little interest in food and health. But why should advice about the best-buy washing machine or toaster be any different from advice about the best-buy apple pie or loaf of bread?

Freedom to choose requires knowledge. If you do not know the difference between good and bad food, you cannot make a reasoned choice. Choice is also distorted by income and availability. Supermarket chains do not want to open up new modern stores in areas of high unemployment. Look at the difference between the supermarkets in rich and poor districts of your own neighbourhood.

We in Britain have been brought up to take about as much interest in food as in the petrol we put in our cars – less, perhaps, since everybody thinks there is a difference between 2-star and 4-star. Children are not taught nutrition in schools. Nutrition is not on the syllabus for doctors, nurses, catering students or supermarket buyers. Government has in the past stated that food is not a health worry. And the British have a habit of taking what they are given, with a grumble, perhaps, but without much question.

Food is an area where the free market does not and cannot operate. The market is and always has been highly manipulated. Subsidies, taxes and allowances, of which the most notorious are the subsidies for fatty meat and milk, affect the price of food all the way along the distribution chain, from seed germination and animal birth, to the plastic pack on the supermarket shelf. Is it right to protect sugar production, but not potatoes or spinach? Or fat meat rather than lean? Or dairy farming rather than the fishing fleet?

The over-riding reason why the free market cannot operate with food is, as has already been stated in this book, that there is, and always will be, a clash between health and wealth, as far as food is concerned. A good food is a bad commodity. Good food goes bad, because it supports life. There is, purely for economic reasons, a constant pressure to drive down the quality of food. To some extent this pressure can be resisted, in a democracy, by consumers insisting on good food and refusing to buy bad food.

But the government does now need to accept a responsibility for a healthy, as well as safe and clean, food supply. This requires laws and regulations governing the quality and composition of food. Explicit labelling, including details of the quantity of saturated fats, sugars, salt and additives in food, is required, simply because we have a right to know what is in the food we eat. But if the consumer is offered four foods, all stating on the label that they contain an additive that the consumer wants to avoid, where is the choice?

We have a right to know what is in the food we eat. We have a right to expect that the food supplied to us is wholesome. And we also have a right to demand an end to the process whereby decisions about the food we eat are taken in secret by people we do not know and do not elect, who sign the Official Secrets Act.

Governments act when there is a practical reason to act. Before the last war the government took a responsibility for a healthy food supply, to ensure that the young men of the nation were fit to fight a war. Until then, the bleak words of John Boyd Orr, written in 1936, applied:

> If children of the three lower groups were reared for profit like young animals, giving them a diet below the requirements for health would be financially unsound. Unfortunately, the health and physical fitness of the rising generation are not marketable commodities which can be assessed in terms of money.

Fifty years later, are Boyd Orr's words true, again? It may be that government will not move until convinced that, without action, the National Health Service will in time collapse under the weight of patients being referred with (often undiagnosed) diet-related diseases. And a bankrupt NHS would, of course, mean a bankrupt nation – physically, morally, and economically.

Eating Well for the Rest of your Life

You can choose to eat well, now. On page 308 are two shopping baskets: the weekly food buys for a family of two adults and two children. The list on the left corresponds to the 'national average' in 1982. The list on the right corresponds to the NACNE goals. You will see that the changes are not dramatic. Some foods are given two stars (**) in the list on the right. These are entirely healthy foods: eat as much as you like of them. The foods with one star (*) are unhealthy foods: the less you eat of these, the better.

The healthy shopping basket is just one of very many you can construct for yourself. The choice here favours lots of fish. You could instead, choose more vegetables and cereals. The overall principle is: eat whole, fresh food, and prefer food of vegetable origin.

A Summary of all the Advice

- FATS Choose oils and margarines, that are high in polyunsaturates (soya, sunflower, safflower, corn, sesame; and also olive). Avoid all other types of artificially hardened (hydrogenated) oils/fats.

- MEAT Choose very lean cuts of beef, lamb, pork, bacon. Eat more poultry, game. Eat pies, tinned meats, sausages, rarely if at all. Go for quality rather than quantity. You do not need animal protein.

- FISH Eat more fish and shellfish of all kinds. Fat fish like herring and mackerel are high in polyunsaturates. Fresh fish are healthier than fish in fatty batter. Find out just how many delicious ways there are of cooking fish.

- DAIRY Buy skimmed or semi-skimmed fresh milk. Use plain yoghurt rather than cream. Have plain yoghurt and fresh fruit rather than 'fruit-flavour' yoghurts. Buy better quality mature cheeses. Don't eat a lot of eggs.

- BREAD Eat lots more good quality wholemeal bread. Have bread at all main meals. Eat sandwiches rather than

	What we eat now †	*What to do*	*The healthy shopping basket*	
BREAD	Mostly white. Some brown.	6¾ lb	more, switch	All wholemeal	13 lb**
FLOUR	White	1¼ lb	switch	Wholemeal, brown	1¼ lb
CAKES, BISCUITS	. . . and pastries, wafers etc.	2½ lb	less, switch	Low fats and sugars	1 lb
BREAKFAST CEREALS	Mostly with sugars and salt	¾ lb	switch	Muesli, no sugars, whole grain	¾ lb**
PASTAS etc.	and rice. White	¼ lb	switch	Wholegrain	¼ lb**
MEAT (FRESH)	Beef, lamb, pork, bacon	4½ lb	less, switch	Lean meat only, more variety	3½ lb
MEAT (PROCESSED)	Sausages, pies, canned meats	2¼ lb	cut out	High quality delicatessen	¼ lb
POULTRY	Almost all chicken	1½ lb	more	More variety	2¼ lb
FISH	Mostly frozen, tinned, fingers	1 lb	much more	Fresh, every variety	4½ lb
POTATOES		8¼ lb	more	New preferably in season	12½ lb
VEGETABLES (OTHER, FRESH)	Mostly carrots, onion, cabbage	5 lb	much more	More variety	12 lb**
VEGETABLES (PROCESSED)	Tinned, frozen beans, peas, chips	3 lb	cut out	Frozen in winter. Dried beans	1 lb**
FRUIT (FRESH)	Mostly apples, oranges, bananas	3½ lb	much more	More variety	9 lb**
FRUIT (PROCESSED)	Tinned and frozen	1½ lb	cut out		
MILK	Almost all full-fat	13½ pt	switch	Semi-skimmed or skimmed	13½ pt
CHEESE	Mostly hard cheeses	¾ lb	switch	Prefer soft cheeses	¾ lb
BUTTER	Mostly salted	¾ lb	less	Prefer unsalted	½ lb*
EGGS		14	less		12
FATS	Mostly soft margarines and lard	1½ lb	less, switch	'High in polyunsaturates' margarine	¾ lb
OILS	Blended vegetable oils	¼ lb	more, switch	High poly. and olive oil	¾ lb
SUGAR (PACKETS)	Almost all white	2½ lb	cut out	Brown is no better	½ lb*
JAMS, PRESERVES	. . . and marmalade, pickles	½ lb	less		¼ lb
SWEETS, CONFECTIONERY	Including chocolate, bars	1½ lb	cut out		¼-½ lb*
DRIED FRUIT, NUTS	With preservatives and salt	¼ lb	more, switch	High quality, no salt (nuts)	¾ lb**

† Household Food Consumption and Expenditure 1982 (MAFF/HMSO 1984)   ** More if you like

* Better still, cut out altogether

greasy pies for lunch. Better quality bread needs less in the way of spreads. Explore whole food shops.

- POTATOES, PASTA, RICE Eat more potatoes, whole, with their skins, but go easy on the butter. Fry chips in polyunsaturated oils. Eat more rice, pasta and noodles. Try wholegrain varieties. Brown rice is easier to cook.

- FRUIT AND VEGETABLES Have fresh fruit instead of puddings or sweet snacks. Try it at breakfast. Eat lots more fresh green vegetables, lightly cooked or in salads. Eat lots more beans and pulses of all varieties.

- BREAKFAST Choose wholegrain breakfast cereals without added sugars or salt. Porridge or muesli are good. Eat them with fresh fruit and with low-fat milks and yoghurts. Eat wholemeal bread, lean bacon.

- SNACKS Fresh and dried fruit and nuts, and sandwiches, are better than 'convenience' biscuits, cakes and confectionery. Scones and teacakes are better than sticky cakes. Avoid all fizzy coloured drinks and colas.

Index

accidents, 57

acne/spots, 56, 284

additives, xxvii, xxviii, xxxvi, 56, 57, 69, 86, 101, 140, 148, 168, 179-81 *passim*, 183, 184, 197, 198, 207, 264, 283-4, 288, 303, 306

  Food Additives and Contaminants Committee, xx

adolescents, 1, 32-5 *passim*, 47, 66, 68

Adulteration, Act for Preventing (1860), 141

advertising, 48, 62, 73, 74, 87-8, 117, 156, 189, 191 195, 233, 249-50, 269, 276, 301, 303, 304

'aerobics', 296-7

Africa, 14, 123, 212, 251, 267, 287

ageing, 20, 33, 59-60, 87

agriculture, xiii, xxii, xxix, 39, 40, 71, 94-5, 100 102, 104, 234-6

  Common Agricultural Policy, 62, 300

  Ministry of, xx, xxi, 12n, 22, 28n, 38, 40, 62, 69, 95, 101, 124-5, 127, 128, 132, 135, 140, 141, 143-5, 183, 196, 220, 237, 238, 240, 242, 259, 262, 263, 302

Aitken, Jonathan, 90, 82, 138

alcohol, xv, xxi, xxxi, 12n 16, 22-5, 35, 36, 38, 39, 48, 53, 54, 56, 58, 100, 177, 217, 274-82, 292, 293

  foetal alcohol syndrome, 56, 281

  'Alcohol Policies', 275-6, 279, 282

alcoholism, 23, 24, 279-80

aldicarb, 263

aldrin, 262, 263

alimentary tract, 53, 55, *see also* gut

All-Bran, 189, 190, 204, 223

allergies, 32, 56, 57, 169, 243, 284

Allied Bakeries, xxvi

Allinson, Dr Thomas, 85-6, 174

aluminium, 60